Andrew Malekoff, MSW
Roselle Kurland, PhD
Editors

A Quarter Century of Classics (1978-2004): Capturing the Theory, Practice, and Spirit of Social Work with Groups

A Quarter Century of Classics (1978-2004): Capturing the Theory, Practice, and Spirit of Social Work with Groups has been co-published simultaneously as *Social Work with Groups*, Volume 28, Numbers 3/4 2005.

*Pre-publication
REVIEWS,
COMMENTARIES,
EVALUATIONS . . .*

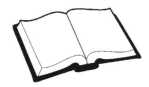

"STUDENTS AND INSTRUCTORS WILL VALUE THIS BOOK TREMEN-DOUSLY. Finally, in one book are several seminal papers on group work theory and practice that have appeared in *Social Work with Groups*. The editors made wise and thoughtful choices; each chapter contributes strongly to the whole. Students of group work, faculty members, and social work scholars will not go wrong by purchasing this text and referring to it in their work. THIS IS A WONDERFUL TEXT!"

Meredith Hanson, DSW
*Director
PhD in Social Work Program
Fordham University Graduate School
of Social Service*

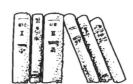

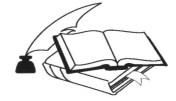

The Haworth Press, Inc.
New York • London

A Quarter Century of Classics (1978-2004): Capturing the Theory, Practice, and Spirit of Social Work with Groups

A Quarter Century of Classics (1978-2004): Capturing the Theory, Practice, and Spirit of Social Work with Groups has been co-published simultaneously as *Social Work with Groups*, Volume 28, Numbers 3/4 2005.

Monographic Separates from *Social Work with Groups*™

For additional information on these and other Haworth Press titles, including descriptions, tables of contents, reviews, and prices, use the QuickSearch catalog at http://www.HaworthPress.com.

A Quarter Century of Classics (1978-2004): Capturing the Theory, Practice, and Spirit of Social Work with Groups, edited by Andrew Malekoff, MSW, and Roselle Kurland, PhD (Vol. 28, No. 3/4, 2005). *A best-of-the-best collection of the most compelling articles published in* Social Work with Groups *since the journal's inception in 1978.*

Stories Celebrating Group Work: It's Not Always Easy to Sit on Your Mouth, edited by Roselle Kurland, PhD, and Andrew Malekoff, ACSW (Vol. 25, No. 1/2, 2002). *"A rare glimpse at some of the crucial moments that have inspired, influenced, and created real groupworkers." (Lainey Collins, CSW, Camp Director, The Fresh Air Fund)*

Support Groups: Current Perspectives on Theory and Practice, edited by Maeda J. Galinsky, PhD, and Janice H. Schopler, PhD (Vol. 18, No. 1, 1996). *"Provides a framework for understanding and examining supportive group interventions. Provides descriptions of different kinds of support groups and alerts practitioners and educators to issues of planning, implementing, and evaluating such services." (The Brown University Child and Adolescent Behavior Newsletter)*

Social Work with Groups: Expanding Horizons, edited by Stanley Wenocur, PhD, Thomas Vassil, PhD, Paul Ephross, PhD, and Raju Varghese, EdD, MPH (Vol. 16, No. 1/2, 1993). *"Fascinating and interesting. The chapters are excellent, spanning theory and direct practice with groups. . . . Helpful to practitioners and educators. I recommend it highly to both." (Joan K. Parry, DSW, LCSW, Professor, College of Social Work, San Jose State University)*

Group Work Reaching Out: People, Places, and Power, edited by James A. Garland, AB, MSSS (Vol. 15, No. 2/3, 1993). *"Experienced leaders in practice and teaching of social work with groups address the problems and potential of a wide variety of vulnerable, alienated, underserved, and politically disenfranchised populations. . . . A must." (Social Work with Groups Newsletter)*

Social Action in Group Work, edited by Abe Vinik and Morris Levin (Vol. 14, No. 3/4, 1992). *"Focuses on getting rid of the causes of problems through group action. . . . Numerous examples are provided for students, educators, researchers, and practitioners." (Social Work with Groups Newsletter)*

Groupwork with Suburbia's Children: Difference, Acceptance, and Belonging, edited by Andrew Malekoff, MSW (Vol. 14, No. 1, 1991). *"Provide[s] a careful, professional look into the multiple problems of the children and youth outside of the inner city and minority areas in which we traditionally expect to find such problems." (Social Work with Groups Newsletter)*

Ethnicity and Biculturalism: Emerging Perspectives of Social Group Work, edited by Kenneth L. Chau, PhD (Vol. 13, No. 4, 1991). *"Offers a tremendous help in focusing on the issues and addresses them in a straightforward manner. It is highly recommended for those in 'helping' professions." (Multiculture Publishers Exchange Newsletter)*

Theory and Practice in Social Group Work: Creative Connections, edited by Marie Weil, DSW, Kenneth L. Chau, PhD, and Dannia Southerland, MSW (Supplement #4, 1991). *Here is an important look at creative ways to successfully blend theoretical knowledge with skillful intervention in social group work.* Theory and Practice in Social Group Work *represents leading works in conceptual development that creatively connect practice with theory and also reflect the current diversity of interventions in group work practice.*

Group Work with the Emotionally Disabled, edited by Baruch Levine, PhD (Vol. 13, No. 1, 1990). *"Provides an excellent overview of group work within a variety of settings and with a variety of populations." (Adult Residential Care Journal)*

Groups in Health Care Settings, edited by Janice H. Schopler, PhD, and Maeda J. Galinsky, PhD (Vol. 12, No. 4, 1990). *"This timely collection offers a broad ranging view of what's happening through groups in hospitals and community agencies." (Ruth R. Middleman, EdD, ACSW, Professor, Kent School of Social Work, University of Louisville)*

Roots and New Frontiers in Social Group Work, by Marcus Leiderman, MSW, Martin L. Birnbaum, PhD, and Barbara Dazzo, PhD (Supplement #3, 1989). *"The vitality of contemporary social group work is reflected in this book. . . . A worthwhile contribution to the literature." (Social Work)*

Social Work with Multi-Family Groups, edited by D. Rosemary Cassano, PhD, MSW (Vol. 12, No. 1, 1989). *Better understand the interrelatedness of the primary family group and the formed therapeutic group with this book.*

Group Work with the Poor and Oppressed, edited by Judith A. B. Lee, DSW (Vol. 11, No. 4, 1989). *"A rich source of reference material for those looking for historical, theoretical, and practical references." (Australian Social Work)*

Violence: Prevention and Treatment in Groups, edited by George S. Getzel, DSW (Vol. 11, No. 3, 1989). *"A useful supplement for a library serving a social work, mental health, or family therapy curriculum." (Academic Library Book Review)*

Social Group Work: Competence and Values in Practice, edited by Joseph Lassner, PhD, MSW, Kathleen Powell, MSW, and Elaine Finnegan, MSW (Supplement #2, 1987). *Detailed information on group work theory, group structure, gender and race issues in group work, group work in health care settings, and the use of groups for coping with family issues that will be invaluable for all professionals in their daily practice.*

Working Effectively with Administrative Groups, edited by Ronald W. Toseland, PhD, and Paul H. Ephross, PhD (Vol. 10, No. 2, 1987). *Exciting suggestions for making administrative groups more effective.*

Collectivity in Social Group Work: Concept and Practice, edited by Norma C. Lang, PhD, and Joanne Sulman, MSW (Vol. 9, No. 4, 1987). *A concise and comprehensive examination of the theory of collectivity in social group work.*

Research in Social Group Work, edited by Sheldon D. Rose, PhD, and Ronald A. Feldman (Vol. 9, No. 3, 1987). *Reflects not only on the important advances and strengths in group work research but also some of the deficiencies and gaps that characterize contemporary research in the field.*

The Legacy of William Schwartz: Group Practice as Shared Interaction, edited by Alex Gitterman, EdD, MSW, and Lawrence Schulman (Vol. 8, No. 4, 1986). *This fine volume celebrates William Schwartz's lasting contribution to teaching and scholarship and conveys the power of his ideas and their relevance to contemporary practice.*

Innovations in Social Group Work: Feedback from Practice to Theory, edited by Marvin Parnes, MSW (Supplement #1, 1986). *This classic volume illustrates just how vigorous and inventive social groupwork can be.*

Time as a Factor in Groupwork: Time-Limited Group Experiences, edited by Albert S. Alissi, DSW, and Max Casper (Vol. 8, No. 2, 1985). *This informative book provides the helping professional with valuable information on the benefits and drawbacks of time-limited social groupwork.*

Groupwork with Children and Adolescents, edited by Ralph L. Kolodny, MA, MSSS, and James A. Garland, ACSW (Vol. 7, No. 4, 1985). *"Integrates time-tested models and procedures with emerging theories and models in a field where a paucity of material exists. . . . Should be of considerable interest to educators as well as social workers." (Voice of Youth Advocates)*

Ethnicity in Social Group Work Practice, edited by Larry E. Davis (Vol. 7, No. 3, 1984). *"Excellent resource. . . . Will serve as a good supplemental text in a generic social group work course or as a main text in a specialized course." (Howard J. Doueck, Social Work Department, State University of New York at Buffalo)*

A Quarter Century of Classics (1978-2004): Capturing the Theory, Practice, and Spirit of Social Work with Groups

Andrew Malekoff, MSW
Roselle Kurland, PhD
Editors

A Quarter Century of Classics (1978-2004): Capturing the Theory, Practice, and Spirit of Social Work with Groups has been co-published simultaneously as *Social Work with Groups*, Volume 28, Numbers 3/4 2005.

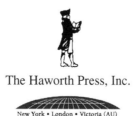

The Haworth Press, Inc.

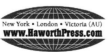

New York • London • Victoria (AU)
www.HaworthPress.com

Published by

The Haworth Press, Inc., 10 Alice Street, Binghamton, NY 13904-1580 USA

A Quarter Century of Classics (1978-2004): Capturing the Theory, Practice, and Spirit of Social Work with Groups has been co-published simultaneously as *Social Work with Groups*, Volume 28, Numbers 3/4 2005.

The development, preparation, and publication of this work has been undertaken with great care. However, the publisher, employees, editors, and agents of The Haworth Press and all imprints of The Haworth Press, Inc., including The Haworth Medical Press® and The Pharmaceutical Products Press®, are not responsible for any errors contained herein or for consequences that may ensue from use of materials or information contained in this work. With regard to case studies, identities and circumstances of individuals discussed herein have been changed to protect confidentiality. Any resemblance to actual persons, living or dead, is entirely coincidental.

The Haworth Press is committed to the dissemination of ideas and information according to the highest standards of intellectual freedom and the free exchange of ideas. Statements made and opinions expressed in this publication do not necessarily reflect the views of the Publisher, Directors, management, or staff of The Haworth Press, Inc., or an endorsement by them.

Cover design by Kerry E. Mack.

Library of Congress Cataloging-in-Publication Data

A quarter century of classics (1978-2004) : capturing the theory, practice, and spirit of social work with groups / Andrew Malekoff, Roselle Kurland, editors.
      p. cm.
   "... co-published simultaneously as Social work with groups, volume 28, numbers 3/4, 2005."
   Includes bibliographical references.
   ISBN-13: 978-0-7890-2872-3 (hard cover : alk. paper)
   ISBN-10: 0-7890-2872-7 (hard cover : alk. paper)
   ISBN-13: 978-0-7890-2873-0 (soft cover : alk. paper)
   ISBN-10: 0-7890-2873-5 (soft cover : alk. paper)
   1. Social group work. 2. Social group work–Case studies. I. Malekoff, Andrew. II. Kurland, Roselle. III. Social work with groups (Haworth Press)

HV45.Q37 2005
361.4–dc22
                              2005033542

Indexing, Abstracting & Website/Internet Coverage

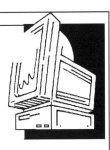

This section provides you with a list of major indexing & abstracting services and other tools for bibliographic access. That is to say, each service began covering this periodical during the year noted in the right column. Most Websites which are listed below have indicated that they will either post, disseminate, compile, archive, cite or alert their own Website users with research-based content from this work. (This list is as current as the copyright date of this publication.)

Abstracting, Website/Indexing Coverage . . . . Year When Coverage Began

- *Academic ASAP <http://www.galegroup.com>* **1994**

- *Academic Search Elite (EBSCO)* **1996**

- *Academic Search Premier (EBSCO)*
  <http://www.epnet.com/academic/acasearchprem.asp> **1996**

- *Applied Social Sciences Index & Abstracts (ASSIA) (Online:*
  ASSI via Data-Star) (CDRom: ASSIA Plus)
  <http://www.csa.com> **1987**

- *Business Source Corporate: coverage of nearly 3,350 quality*
  magazines and journals; designed to meet the diverse information
  needs of corporations; EBSCO Publishing <http://www.epnet.com/
  corporate/bsourcecorp.asp> **1996**

- *CareData: the database supporting social care management*
  and practice <http://www.elsc.org.uk/caredata/caredata.htm> . . . **1975**

- *CINAHL (Cumulative Index to Nursing & Allied Health Literature),*
  in print, EBSCO, and SilverPlatter, DataStar, and PaperChase.
  (Support materials include Subject Heading List, Database Search
  Guide, and instructional video) <http://www.cinahl.com> **2003**

- *e-psyche, LLC <http://www.e-psyche.net>* **2001**

- *EBSCOhost Electronic Journals Service (EJS)*
  <http://ejournals.ebsco.com> **2001**

(continued)

(continued)

(continued)

Special Bibliographic Notes related to special journal issues (separates) and indexing/abstracting:

- indexing/abstracting services in this list will also cover material in any "separate" that is co-published simultaneously with Haworth's special thematic journal issue or DocuSerial. Indexing/abstracting usually covers material at the article/chapter level.
- monographic co-editions are intended for either non-subscribers or libraries which intend to purchase a second copy for their circulating collections.
- monographic co-editions are reported to all jobbers/wholesalers/approval plans. The source journal is listed as the "series" to assist the prevention of duplicate purchasing in the same manner utilized for books-in-series.
- to facilitate user/access services all indexing/abstracting services are encouraged to utilize the co-indexing entry note indicated at the bottom of the first page of each article/chapter/contribution.
- this is intended to assist a library user of any reference tool (whether print, electronic, online, or CD-ROM) to locate the monographic version if the library has purchased this version but not a subscription to the source journal.
- individual articles/chapters in any Haworth publication are also available through the Haworth Document Delivery Service (HDDS).

I dedicate this collection of classic group work articles to the memory of my friend, colleague and fellow editor Roselle Kurland (1943-2005).

Andrew Malekoff

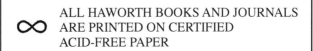

ABOUT THE EDITORS

Andrew Malekoff, MSW, is Associate Executive Director of the North Shore Child and Family Guidance Center in Roslyn Heights, New York, where he has worked since 1977. He is a widely published author and an internationally known lecturer. His most recent book is the second edition of the critically acclaimed *Group Work with Adolescents: Principles and Practice*, a main selection of the Behavioral Science Book Club. Mr. Malekoff has taught as Adjunct Professor at Adelphi University, serves on the board of directors of the Association for the Advancement of Social Work with Groups, and is consulting editor for several professional journals.

Roselle Kurland, PhD, (1943-2005) was Professor at the Hunter College School of Social Work. She co-authored both the third edition of the text *Social Work with Groups* (with Helen Northen) and *Teaching a Methods Course in Social Work with Groups* (with Robert Salmon). She was involved with group work practice, training, and consultation with a wide variety of social work agencies and organizations. Dr. Kurland was co-editor of the journal *Social Work with Groups* (with Andrew Malekoff) from 1990 until her death in 2005.

A Quarter Century
of Classics
(1978-2004):
Capturing the Theory,
Practice, and Spirit
of Social Work with Groups

CONTENTS

ABOUT THE AUTHORS

Margot Breton, MSW, is Professor Emerita, Faculty of Social Work, University of Toronto. Address correspondence to 160 Rosedale Heights Drive, Toronto, Ontario M4T 1C8, Canada (margotbreton@sympatico. ca). At the time her article appeared she was on the faculty of University of Toronto.

Allan Brown, DSA, is an olive farmer in southern Greece. Address correspondence to Tseria, Kardamyli 24022, Messinia, Greece (celliala@ otenet.gr). At the time his article appeared, he was Senior Lecturer, School of Applied Social Studies, University of Briston, England.

Marcia B. Cohen, PhD, is Professor, University of New England, School of Social Work. Address correspondence to 716 Stevens Avenue, Portland, ME 04193 (mcohen@une.edu). At the time her article appeared, she was Associate Professor at the University of New England School of Social Work.

Trudy K. Duffy, PhD. At the time her article appeared she was Clinical Professor, Boston University School of Social Work. Address correspondence to Colcord Pond Road, Porter, ME 04068.

Maeda J. Galinsky, MSW, PhD, is Kenan Distinguished Professor, University of North Carolina at Chapel Hill, 301 Pittsboro Street, CB#3550, Chapel Hill, NC 27599-3550 (maeda@email.unc.edu). At the time her article appeared she was Assistant Professor at UNC.

Alex Gitterman, MSW, EdD, is Professor, School of Social Work, University of Connecticut, 1798 Asylum Avenue, West Hartford, CT 06117 (Alex.Gitterman@uconn.edu). At the time his article appeared, he was Professor, Columbia University School of Social Work.

Margaret E. Hartford, PhD, died in April, 2003. At the time her article appeared, she was Professor of Gerontology and Social Work, Leonard David School of Gerontology, Andrus Center, University of Southern California.

Jana Jagendorf, MSW, is Social Work of the Litchfield School District, 1 Highlander Court, Litchfield, NH 03052 (Jjagendorf@litchfieldsd.org). At the time her article appeared, she was Social Worker, Intensive Support Program, North Shore Child and Family Guidance Center.

Gisela Konopka, DSW, died in December 2003. At the time her article appeared, she was Director, University of Minnesota Center for Youth Development and Research.

Roselle Kurland, PhD, died in June, 2005. At the time this collection was being developed she was Professor, Hunter College School of Social Work. At the time her article on planning appeared, she was a doctoral student at the University of Southern California. At the time her article on group work vs. casework in a group appeared, she was Associate Professor at Hunter.

Andrew Malekoff, MSW, is Associate Director, North Shore Child and Family Guidance Center, Roslyn Heights, NY 11577 (amalekoff@ northshorechildguidance.org). At the time his article appeared, he was Director of Program Development at that agency.

Ruth Middleman, EdD, died in March 2005. At the time her article appeared, she was Professor, Raymond A. Kent School of Social Work, University of Louisville.

Rachel Miller, MSW, is Senior Research Social Worker, Zucker Hillside Hospital, 75-79 263 Street, Glen Oaks, NY 11004 (rmilles@ optonline.net). At the time her article appeared she was Senior Social Worker at that Hospital.

Tara Mistry, DASS, CQSW, is Consultant (Health and Social Care), Munsad Consultancy and Research, 115A, Birchwood Road, Briston, BS4 4RB, England (taramistry@btopenworld.com). At the time her article appeared, she was Lecturer in Social Work, School of Applied Social Studies, University of Bristol.

Audrey Mullender, PhD, is Principal, Ruskin College, and Professor in Social Work, University of Warwick. Address correspondence to Ruskin College, Walton Street, Oxford, OX1 2HE, UK (amullender@ruskin.ac.uk). At the time her article appeared, she was Professor, University of Warwick, Department of Applied Social Sciences, Warwick, England.

Robert Salmon, DSW, is Professor, Hunter College School of Social Work, 129 East 79 Street, New York, NY 10021 (rssalmon@rcn.com). At the time his article appeared he was Professor, Hunter College.

Erica Schnekenburger, MSW, was unable to be located at the time of publication. At the time her article appeared, she was Clinical Social Worker, Family and Children's Services of Maryland.

Janice Schopler, PhD, died in December 1999. At the time her article appeared, she was Assistant Professor, School of Social Work, University of North Carolina at Chapel Hill.

William Schwartz, died in August, 1982. This article was published in a special issue of the Journal, "The Legacy of William Schwartz: Group Practice as Shared Interaction," that was published soon after his death.

Dominique Moyse Steinberg, DSW, is Assistant Professor, Hunter College School of Social Work. Address correspondence to 1 Lincoln Plaza, New York, NY 10023 (dmsvt@earthlink.net). At the time her article appeared, she was Adjunct Instructor, Hunter College School of Social Work.

Whitney Wright, CSW, is Founder and Director of Keep it in the Ring, 962 Carolina Street, San Francisco, CA 94101 (whitwrigt@rcn.com). At the time her article appeared, she was Youth Specialist, The Family Center, New York, NY.

Preface

Developing a collection of "classic" articles that have appeared in *Social Work with Groups* over a quarter century plus has been a daunting task. We began the process by writing to members of our editorial board asking for their recommendations. We defined "classic" as articles that have had a significant impact on group work theory and practice, articles that have been memorable and useful, and articles that meet any or all of the following criteria:

- Articles that have been particularly useful to students' practice over the years as reflected in their papers, practice logs, and classroom contributions;
- Articles that have advanced theory, adding significantly to the conceptual foundation of group work practice; and
- Articles that have best captured the heart and spirit of group work through vivid illustrations and/or reflections on practice that are conceptually sound.

We reviewed the responses and organized them by frequency of recommendation and included our own suggestions in the mix. Then we reviewed each of the articles. It was our hope that the recommendations would be representative of the 1970s, 1980s, 1990s, and 2000s and would include articles written by individuals working in the classroom and in the field.

One of the things that made the task most daunting was that we knew from the beginning that we would be bound to neglect some important

[Haworth co-indexing entry note]: "Preface." Malekoff, Andrew, and Roselle Kurland. Co-published simultaneously in *Social Work with Groups* (The Haworth Press, Inc.) Vol. 28, No. 3/4, 2005, pp. xxvii-xxix; and: *A Quarter Century of Classics (1978-2004): Capturing the Theory, Practice, and Spirit of Social Work with Groups* (ed: Andrew Malekoff, and Roselle Kurland) The Haworth Press, Inc., 2005, pp. xxiii-xxv. Single or multiple copies of this article are available for a fee from The Haworth Document Delivery Service [1-800-HAWORTH, 9:00 a.m. - 5:00 p.m. (EST). E-mail address: docdelivery@haworthpress.com].

xxiii

articles that could not be fit in due to limitations of space. After all, we were considering more than 100 issues of the Journal with some 600 articles. In fact, we approached the publisher early on with a proposal for a triple issue of the Journal rather than double one so that additional articles could be incorporated. Triple issues are not feasible for marketing, nor are they advisable for meeting the needs of subscribers who expect four journal issues per year. We even wondered whether we made the right decision to produce such a collection, knowing in advance that there would be repercussions. It must be obvious, however, if you are reading this, that we decided that it was the right decision to move ahead.

We have thoughtfully and painstakingly selected a wonderful and representative collection that fits the criteria as stated above and that reflects the theory, practice and spirit of social work with groups over the past quarter century. We do expect to be hearing from our readers and authors who will ask us "How could you not have included . . . ?" We may have overlooked a favorite article of yours or one that you have written that appeared in the Journal. Although it will be difficult to hear about what articles were overlooked, it will please us to know that for over twenty-five years our readers have found so many articles worthy of the designation of "classic" that we were unable to fit them all into this edition.

In the end, we chose articles that covered themes including planning, ethics, mutual aid, race, gender, time, social reform, program, and metaphor. We included articles that addressed practice with the young and old, struggling with a range of needs, and in a variety of settings. We took special care to include articles that included some of the more moving and well developed examples of group work in action, as we are always concerned as editors that we integrate the theoretical and descriptive by wedding concepts and illustrations into the articles we choose, the volumes we produce.

The seventeen articles in this volume begin with the very first article in the very first issue of the Journal published in the spring of 1978 under the leadership of founding editors Catherine Papell and Beulah Rothman. Their choice to inaugurate the Journal with Margaret E. Hartford's *Groups in the Human Services: Some Facts and Fancies* is one that we now repeat in this issue of classics. The collection then wends its way through the next four decades, ending with Rachel Miller's 2002 essay *Will the Real Healer Please Take a Bow*, that appeared in a collection of stories that we edited celebrating the Journal's twenty-fifth anniversary. Perhaps her's is a fitting title with which to end this volume, by prompting *Social Work with Groups*, on behalf of all of its authors and readers to take a well-deserved bow.

Andrew Malekoff
Roselle Kurland (1943-2005)
Editors

Groups in the Human Services:
Some Facts and Fancies

Margaret E. Hartford

SUMMARY. Many misconceptions are associated with the use of groups in social work practice, especially by those practitioners who do not have a grasp of small group theory and leadership methods and skills. Historically, social workers have believed that collective behavior could change attitudes, give participants a sense of support and belonging, develop new knowledge, socialize behavior, and influence systems and organizations. The growing body of small group research, and research on practice with groups in social work and other professions, can remove some of the mystery and make possible more deliberate and definitive use of groups. Furthermore, a worker needs a commitment to values in the use of groups, and a grasp of the dynamics of helping the participants to make use of their group relationships to achieve their goals. We have the knowledge and skill at our fingertips to provide an instrument which many people in society are seeking. *[Article copies available for a fee from The Haworth Document Delivery Service: 1-800-HAWORTH. E-mail address: <docdelivery@haworthpress.com> Website: <http://www.HaworthPress.com> © 2005 by The Haworth Press, Inc. All rights reserved.]*

Dr. Hartford is Professor of Gerontology and Social Work, Leonard Davis School of Gerontology, Andrus Center, University of Southern California, Los Angeles, CA 90007.

This paper is adapted from an address to Los Amigos de Hurnidad Support Group of the School of Social Work, University of Southern California, Los Angeles.

This article was originally published in *Social Work with Groups*, Vol. 1 (1) © 1978 by The Haworth Press, Inc.

[Haworth co-indexing entry note]: "Groups in the Human Services: Some Facts and Fancies." Hartford, Margaret E. Co-published simultaneously in *Social Work with Groups* (The Haworth Press, Inc.) Vol. 28, No. 3/4, 2005, pp. 1-8; and: *A Quarter Century of Classics (1978-2004): Capturing the Theory, Practice, and Spirit of Social Work with Groups* (ed: Andrew Malekoff, and Roselle Kurland) The Haworth Press, Inc., 2005, pp. 1-8. Single or multiple copies of this article are available for a fee from The Haworth Document Delivery Service [1-800-HAWORTH, 9:00 a.m. - 5:00 p.m. (EST). E-mail address: docdelivery@haworthpress.com].

doi:10.1300/J009v28n03_01

Because of the kinds of things which can happen to people *in* groups–or the things which can happen *as the result of groups*–there is sometimes a great sense of mystery and magic about groups, or even the belief that groups all unto themselves can work miracles, or that if you just bring people together for a group something great will happen. This is only partly true. While groups have power to heal, to nurture, to develop, to educate–they also have the power to destroy their members and those outside. And usually groups do not just happen. They take deliberate work on the part of both leadership and membership.

It has become obvious to social workers that there is a rapidly expanding extension of the uses of groups in all of the human services. The decade of the 1960s has been referred to as the period in which social workers discovered and rediscovered the group. Not only did we discover that there were some personal and social needs and problems of individuals that responded better to group methods, but we also rediscovered the political force and power of organization and collective action in community efforts for system management and change.

The social democrats and adult educators of the 1920s–Lindemann (1924), Harrison Elliot (1928), Coyle (1930, 1937), and Shieffield (1922, 1929)–the trade unionists, the settlement workers in ethnic neighborhoods, the feminists first time around–knew the value of collective behavior for changing attitudes, for helping people gain a sense of belonging, for developing new knowledge, for socializing behavior, but also for bringing about societal and institutional change. And the designers of the youth movements, Ys, Scouts, and Boys' and Girls' Clubs, had some ideas about the meaning of belonging for influencing values and behavior of the young. All of these streams of goal-directed group use–or purposeful development of groups for specific objectives–laid the foundations for present-day group uses.

Yet, today many people are seizing upon the group as an instrument for help or change, action and growth, as if the group were newly invented. People are picking up techniques and gimmicks–which may lead to good or to questionable results with people in groups–but without the theoretical underpinnings to understand why they are using these methods or what may be the potential outcomes. Activities that we engaged in as parlor games and icebreakers when we were kids have been legitimized into group techniques, such as the blind walk, games of trust, or feeling and touching–and a couple we called "sardines" and "post office." They *do* encourage interaction.

There is a growing body of knowledge about small group behavior (Hare, 1976), based not only on hunches and armchair theory development and upon findings of experimental collectivities of individuals convened for research, but also empirical research on groups constructed for treatment, help, growth, change, and self-management. *The Journal of Group Psychotherapy* is full of reports on such researches, and Lieberman, Yallom, and Miles (1973) have presented a substantial study, *Encounter Groups: First Facts*, which appeared in *Psychology Today* and now has appeared in a book, a carefully documented piece of research. They found through an extensive study of various types of encounter groups that simply getting people to feel or to act out in a group did not bring about change in people, but rather group members needed help cognitively to gain insight. Analyzing what had taken place and reflecting on it brought more lasting benefits (something we have used in both individual and group work for some time in social work). They also found that expressing anger in groups may be more dysfunctional than helpful, may drive people from groups and be personally destructive–and that people seem to learn better, grow and change more in an atmosphere of love and support.

There seems to be an increasing use of groups on an experiential level, without benefit of the available knowledge. One of my esteemed colleagues on the East Coast who is a well-known practitioner, writer, and teacher said to me recently, "You know there is no theory of small groups. The only way you can learn about groups is experientially–by being in one–learning by trial and error." His view is shared by many. I think that there may be a growing gap between the existing knowledge that is available to us for deliberate and definitive use and the experiential or feeling action and reaction that it is "just good to get people together in a group and something helpful will happen with little guidance or leadership."

Another myth is that if a worker collects an aggregate, that is, gets people together in the same place, and responds to them individually in the presence of each other, something significant and helpful will occur. It may and it may not. It may be good and it may be harmful for individuals in a gathering to observe a therapist responding to one and then another in sequence, but it is not working with the group and it is not maximizing the full potential of having the group begin to work for itself. It is rather doing what I call "aggregational therapy of individuals."

Let me clarify: by the concept *group* I am referring to two or more (and usually more) people interacting with and reacting to each other in such a way as to have meaning for each other and influence over each other, and developing a sense of uniqueness about the relationships that sets this collectivity apart from all other collective relationships of the people who are a part of it (the traditional sociological definition) (Hartford, 1971). This definition does not, therefore, cover people together in the same room unless something is happening among them–some sense of "we" developing.

Let me cite some examples of what I mean by the use of theory to improve practice with groups. Extensive research on spontaneous and autonomous groups, as well as on groups that have been specifically collected for particular purposes, suggests that all groups go through a series of phases in their development from the moment they are convened for the first time and engage in certain social rituals and pastimes–from their initial formation process, through one or several storming periods, on to getting to work on both the *content* for which they were convened and the *development of the group* itself, to planning for termination and the final termination (Tuckman, 1965). While these phases seem to be inevitable in some form in all groups, knowledge of their existence, and the kinds of individual and interpersonal behavior that may occur in each of the phases, provides a worker with some guide to his interventions and activities with the collection of people or with individuals at given points in the group life cycle (Northen, 1968).

Furthermore, knowledge of certain group processes and their interrelatedness may give a worker more skill in helping the group to become a viable instrument for help or change. For instance, the worker's proactive behavior in composition (if there is a choice of deciding who should participate) related to agency or worker service objectives for the group, and related to decisions about frequency, duration, and size, and determining possible individual participants' expectations for the group, may lead to a more compatible group entity. A group may coalesce more rapidly and get to work on achieving that which it was set up to do (whether therapy, task achievement, or system change). That is, if we anticipate and plan for goal-directed activity, think through to the possible end, we may be able to convene a group with a fairly clear contract, and help it to form and then let it flow toward goals that are compatible with the expectations of all participants.

Or if we use theory to think about co-leadership, co-therapy, or team teaching for that matter, we must recognize that we are introducing into the group a two-person subgroup which must be dealt with by all of the participants, as well as by the co-therapists themselves in order to construct a productive group form.

We may choose to have an open-ended group that has a constant turnover in membership. While it is the most effective form (or only possible form) in some settings, this means that the group will have low cohesion and experience some storming each time it adds or loses membership, and that the worker will have to remain fairly central and provide continuity.

For all these examples just stated, there has been enough research and theory development for us to be more and more definitive about our worker activity in using groups (Hartford, 1971).

We are living in an era when groups are being used for or are credited with a great many kinds of human endeavor. The great wave of sensitivity groups, swinging singles, swinging couples, nude workshops, drug drop-in center groups, lay therapy marital couples groups makes us alert to the phenomenon that is sweeping the country. People are seeking personal involvement and belonging of greater depth through various types of group forms. People of all ages–but especially youth, young adults, and older adults or aged–are reaching out, and group solutions are being sought for various kinds of relationship needs. People subjected to computers, social distance, and faceless communications media are reaching for a personalized response through some type of group experience. People automated into stereotyped roles and surrounded by chrome, glass, and concrete are trying to find warmth, personal worth, and affectionate involvement in groups. Perhaps this is a substitute for the extended family of the past.

On the other hand, well-heeled and well-educated youngish middle-aged men testify at Senate hearings that they were led to engage in subversive and criminal acts because it was part of the culture of their group. They trusted their leader and their friends, and it was more important to be somebody in the group than to follow individual values (Dean, 1976). (Didn't we get this message from the street gang members a decade ago?) (Spergel, 1966). And the young people who got involved with Manson and committed crimes justified their behavior as part of the group activity and belonging to "the family." The young political participants testified that they learned their "dirty tricks" in campus organized politics (*West Side Story* in button-down collars). These facts make us pause to give some thought to the care that we must take in our deliberate use of groups as the instrument of help, growth, change, rehabilitation, and social action, social change, and community development. A group can become a tremendous force on its members. The group experience can influence its members even when they have left the presence–for if it has been well formed the socializing effect causes the members to carry group values, norms, and influence with them wherever they go. The group can also carry strong weight in society.

Those very elements in groups which can be positive and helpful may also be destructive and harmful to individuals and to society. So we need all of the knowledge that we can get, and we need to use it with planning, carefully and thoughtfully within the value framework that characterizes our profession. We need to examine the ethics of influence, and the goals or outcomes of our planned behavior with people in groups.

In our eagerness to get onto the group bandwagon, for whatever reason, we must become knowledgeable about group processes to make sure that our groups are helpful and useful, and not destructive or employed irresponsibly or outside of the context of values and skills which characterize social work. We have, for instance, values about the integrity of each individual, his right to expression along with his responsibility for the others in his interactions, his right to privacy and confidentiality so that he is made aware of the risks of some of his expressions in groups, his right to his defenses until he has better ways of protecting himself, his right to self-determination of the direction in which he goes so long as he is not destructive to others and to himself. Our common sense tells us (if we don't have the group theory to support it) that group contagion and group influence may cause people to expose their inner feelings or to act out in ways that are not helpful to themselves in the long run, that may harm others, and that may later be regretted. Some of the techniques in use with groups today (hopefully not in social work) would give sanction to such behaviors without a sense of responsibility to the person in or after the group. The social worker who is committed to his professional ethics must assume some responsibility for the behaviors in which he encourages the group to engage, and must use methods deliberately to facilitate and help the participants. He assumes some responsibility to help members when taking action about a faulty system or institution to present full knowledge that such action may bring on retaliatory effects. The social worker helps an activist group to have some foresight about the possible or inevitable reaction to their activity in order that they be prepared for the consequences when they make a decision to act. The social worker is aware of the resocializing effect and the influence which a group may have on its members, and is therefore aware that while a group can be an anchor and support to help a person to change some of his behavior for positive ends–such as breaking bad habits or kicking addictions–the same phenomenon may offer support to engage in delinquency–or result in brainwashing, or push toward undesirable conformity.

I would submit that just as there is an increasing body of knowledge which all social workers need to have about individual personality theory within its sociocultural context–and new methodologies for maximizing the human potential through various individual helping modalities and new knowledge about systems, societies, and communities–there is also a growing body of knowledge about small groups, their process, and the functioning of individuals in them, and various new methodologies for maximizing human potential and maximizing societal functioning through group processes. I have a growing concern about what we are not teaching social work students or not putting into staff development in our agencies as we encourage all social workers to use group methods. Speaking as one who has been instrumental in curriculum development at a school of social work and who teaches in the human behavior sequence, I am afraid that we are reducing the content about small group processes *by default* as we increase theory about individuals, families, social systems, and organizations–and have left small group theory as an elective. Furthermore, I was chairman of the development of social work practice methods sequence where we put together content on working with individuals, families, and communities through individual and group methods, and I have great concern that we are lessening the amount of knowledge we are teaching about small groups and some of the value questions about using group methods, just at the moment when we are expecting all social workers to use more group methods for work with individuals, families, institutions, and communities. I am puzzled at the inconsistency of our beliefs, behaviors, and expectations, and my only explanation for it is that we may ourselves be guilty of thinking that groups have a mystique and a magic, and that people brought together will somehow form themselves into a helping and helpful entity to work miracles for each other. Or else, perhaps we fail to understand the concept of group, and have not yet integrated our practice and our theory.

It is a fact that groups can and do exist, that there is a body of knowledge that can be understood, and that understanding this knowledge can lead to planned and deliberate behavior on the part of the social worker, who, carrying the ethics of his profession and the values regarding the outcomes of service, can help to construct groups for the benefit of the participants, and groups in which the participants are working to benefit society, community, or mankind. This is not a myth, nor a fancy. And the reality is that studied, proactive and active behavior by the social worker, based on knowledge, can provide him an instrument with a potential beyond what he has yet dreamed.

Groups as a means of social work service delivery, within almost every context–schools, hospitals, family counseling, child welfare, institutions, community services for the elderly, neighborhood organization, community planning–offer us a rare and valuable opportunity (Schwartz & Zalba, 1971). If we understand the resource we have, it will not be a fancy or a myth but a fact and a reality, a greater resource in helping people. The knowledge is there–we have but to reach for it, and to incorporate it into our practice and our teaching. And all over our society people are searching for an instrument which we have at our fingertips. Our responsibility is to make it available and to use it in our administration, our staff relations, our service delivery, and to keep people attached to something that has meaning and can be used as well to perpetuate a free society.

REFERENCES

Coyle. G. *Social process in organized groups*. New York: R. R. Smith, 1930.

Coyle, G. *Studies in group behavior*. New York: Harper, 1937.

Dean, F. *Blind ambition*. New York: Simon and Schuster, 1976.

Elliott, H. S. *The process of group thinking*. New York: Association Press, 1928.

Hare, A. P. *Handbook of small group research* (2nd ed.). New York: Free Press, 1976.

Hartford, M. E. *Groups in social work: Applications of small group research to social work practice*. New York: Columbia Press, 1971.

Leiberman, M., Yallom, I., & Miles, M. *Encounter groups: First facts*. New York: Basic Books, 1973.

Lindemann, E. *Social discovery*. New York: Republic, 1924.

Northen, H. *Social work with groups*. New York: Columbia University Press, 1968.

Schwartz, W., & Zalba, S. *The practice of group work*. New York: Columbia University Press, 1971.

Sheffield, A. D. *Joining in public discussion*. New York: Doran, 1922.

Sheffield, A. D. *Training for group experience*. New York: The Inquiry, 1929.

Spergel, I. *Street gang work: Theory and practice*. Reading, Mass.: Addison-Wesley, 1966.

Tuckman, B. Developmental sequence in small groups. *Psychological Bulletin*, 1965, 63, 384-399.

Planning:
The Neglected Component
of Group Development

Roselle Kurland

SUMMARY. This article identifies pregroup planning–the thinking and preparation done by the social worker in developing a group program–as a neglected area of social work practice. Though the importance of planning is recognized by many writers, little is said about the planning process itself that can help direct and guide the thinking of the social work practitioner. Possible reasons for this gap in our literature and practice are presented. Development of a model of planning for group practice is called for. Components of such a model are drawn from social work writings on work with groups and from research, and a tentative model is suggested. *[Article copies available for a fee from The Haworth Document Delivery Service: 1-800-HAWORTH. E-mail address: <docdelivery@haworthpress.com> Website: <http://www.HaworthPress.com> © 2005 by The Haworth Press, Inc. All rights reserved.]*

Ms. Kurland, a doctoral candidate at the University of Southern California School of Social Work, is former program director of University Settlement in New York City.

This article was originally published in *Social Work with Groups*, Vol. 1 (2) © 1978 by The Haworth Press, Inc.

[Haworth co-indexing entry note]: "Planning: The Neglected Component of Group Development." Kurland, Roselle. Co-published simultaneously in *Social Work with Groups* (The Haworth Press, Inc.) Vol. 28, No. 3/4, 2005, pp. 9-16; and: *A Quarter Century of Classics (1978-2004): Capturing the Theory, Practice, and Spirit of Social Work with Groups* (ed: Andrew Malekoff, and Roselle Kurland) The Haworth Press, Inc., 2005, pp. 9-16. Single or multiple copies of this article are available for a fee from The Haworth Document Delivery Service [1-800-HAWORTH, 9:00 a.m. - 5:00 p.m. (EST). E-mail address: docdelivery@haworthpress.com].

doi:10.1300/J009v28n03_02

Planning for group practice is one of the most neglected areas in social work with groups. The thinking and preparation done by the social worker in undertaking to offer group service too often consists only of cursory attention to such questions as meeting place and time and whether to serve refreshments.

The price for lack of thorough and thoughtful planning is high. Frequently, it is paid in groups that terminate prematurely, groups in which attendance of members is sporadic and irregular, and groups that are felt by practitioners and group members to have failed in meeting the needs of group members. It is paid also in a lack of worker confidence that results in practitioners who shy away from working with groups because they see themselves as incapable of group leadership.

The importance of planning in social work practice with groups, as well as with individuals and families, is recognized by many writers. Some of the profession's most basic definitions include planning as an important social work activity. Bartlett (1958), for example, in the working definition of social work, states: "Social work method includes systematic observation and assessment of the individual or group in a situation and the formulation of an appropriate plan of action" (p. 7). Boehm (1958) considers planning one of four core activities in social work. The importance of pregroup planning is stated most directly by Brody (1974):

> *The most important activities of a worker engaged in group work with institutionalized older adults (as with all clients) are those that occur before any formalized meeting with group members ever takes place. . . . The worker activities that often get the least attention and which are the most crucial to the outcome of the program are related to the thinking, planning, and preparation that occurs prior to the convening of any meeting.* (pp. 125-126)

But, while the importance of planning in social work is recognized, little is said about the planning process itself that can help direct and guide the thinking of the social work practitioner before he initiates direct service with groups. The lack of content on pregroup planning represents a serious gap in social work literature, and it is this gap that may be one of the reasons for the paucity of attention to planning by social work practitioners.

A possible explanation for the lack of attention paid to planning is offered by Dewey (1938), whose writings significantly influenced social group work practice. Writing on progressive education, Dewey explains that weakness in control in the classroom most often goes back to lack of "sufficiently thoughtful planning in advance" (p. 57). He then explains, "The causes for such lack are varied. The one which is peculiarly important to mention . . . is the idea that such advance planning is unnecessary and even that it is inherently hostile to the legitimate freedom of those being instructed" (p. 57). Dewey goes on to say:

> *Because the kind of advance planning heretofore engaged in has been so routine as to leave little room for the free play of individual thinking or for contributions due to distinctive individual experience, it does not follow that all planning must be rejected. On the contrary, there is incumbent upon the educator the duty of instituting a much more intelligent and consequently more difficult kind of planning. He must survey the capacities and needs of the particular set of individuals with whom he is dealing and must at the same time arrange the conditions which provide the subject matter or content for experiences that satisfy these needs and develop these capacities. The planning must be flexible enough to permit free play for individuality of experience and yet firm enough to give direction towards continuous development of power.* (p. 58)

Dewey's words seem equally applicable to social work as to education.

Rosenthal (1973) offers a similar explanation for the lack of attention to the planning phase in work with groups. He states:

> *The artificial group has been recognized in social group work in the expression* formed group, *but the implications of* formed *in terms of artificiality or creation by design have not been explored. . . . One reason for these blind spots is that the directiveness and subjective desire that seem inescapable from the deliberateness involved in forming a group . . . are considered negative. They are regarded as being close to manipulation, and manipulation must be avoided at all costs in social work.* (p. 61)

Rosenthal's explanation may be correct. Perhaps the lack of attention to pre-group planning results from the social work profession's emphasis on client self-determination. Perhaps planning has been viewed as client manipulation and hence as a negation of this important social work value. But one could certainly argue that pregroup planning does not diminish, but instead enhances, the opportunities for client self-determination. The increased clarity of purpose for the social work practitioner and the client that results from careful planning increases the client's ability to make a clear and informed decision about whether he wishes to participate in the service offered and thus lessens client manipulation and domination by the worker and increases client self-determination.

The National Association of Social Workers' (1964) publication *Building Social Work Knowledge* offers another clue as to the possible reasons for the lack of attention paid to planning in the social work literature. Social workers, the publication notes, are more interested in action than in developing and testing knowledge to make that action more effective. Perhaps social workers too often equate helping with "busy-ness" and see the amount of help as being in direct proportion to the amount of activity of the worker. Perhaps planning is viewed as a rather "passive" activity, one that takes time away from the real and "active" work that is done directly with clients. Perhaps in their haste to "get busy," social work practitioners and writers as well have too often cut short the planning process or aborted it altogether.

Development of a model of planning for social work with groups would be an important first step in filling this gap that exists in both our literature and our practice. Such a model would help guide the thinking of the social work practitioner regarding group formation and would furnish needed practice knowledge in this area by providing requisite conceptualization of the planning process.

Clues as to the components of a pregroup planning model are present in social work writing and research. Although there is a paucity of writing on social work practice that addresses planning directly, some authors write about areas that might form components of a planning model. See, for example, Bernstein, 1973a, 1973b; Glasser, Sarri, & Vinter, 1974; Levine, 1967.) Of the writers on social work with groups, for example, Northen (1969) and Hartford (1971) include the most comprehensive material on planning. Northen's work includes the components of purpose, group composition, initial organizational structure, application and intake, and social diagnosis as elements to be considered in planning. Hartford explicates a "pregroup phase" and states:

> *Who makes the decision to have a group, the suggested purposes of the projected group, decisions about who should be informed that there might be a group, and how they are to be informed or selected, and by whom, has a great deal of effect on what happens later when an actual group comes into being.* (p. 70)

Hartford sees group purpose, program, composition, size and meeting place, space, time, and duration as interdependent and interrelated factors that must be thought through by the worker.

No social work research has been carried out on comprehensive planning for direct practice. But consideration has been given in research to some of the elements that might form part of a model of planning for social work with groups. These include clarity of purpose; individual and group goals; group composition and membership selection; client expectations of social work service; and individual diagnoses.

Garvin's (1968) research on complementarity of role expectations in groups between worker and members includes many implications for pregroup planning. Garvin emphasizes the need for early knowledge on the worker's part about member goals and expectations. Such knowledge, he states, is important because it helps the worker to better understand member-worker interaction, indicates how unified the group will be in attempting to solve problems, and offers clues about the degree to which a given member will be invested in pursuing different kinds of group goals. According to Garvin, the social worker's correct perception of members' expectations leads to more skillful worker performance and movement in group problem solving.

Garvin also stresses the importance of clarity of goals. He states:

> *For too long, the assumption has been made in much of group work service planning that the group can and should represent a "smorgasbord" in which virtually any need of the members can be met so long as the necessary requirement of group attendance is maintained.* (p. 201)

Current thinking, he explains, places more emphasis on a precondition of clarity of goals as a means of goal achievement.

Garvin's research thus indicates that early knowledge of member goals and expectations as well as clarity of goals should be included in a pregroup planning model.

Research on client expectations also has important implications for a pregroup planning model. It shows the need for the worker to have early information regarding client expectations, and points to the importance of congruity of expectations between worker and client. Briar (1966) notes, "There is strong evidence, both from casework and psychotherapy research, that clients are more apt to continue in treatment when they and their therapists share similar expectations" (pp. 25-26).

Main's (1964) research on the beginning phase of social group work also contain implications for a model of planning for social work with groups. She concluded that the degree of development of individual and group diagnoses, treatment goals, and plans were positively associated with the degree of appropriateness of the worker's use of self with a group.

Main also raises an important question regarding the connection between planning and diagnosis. She asks, "If practice theory more clearly defined and refined the process of preliminary treatment planning . . . would individual treatment goals and plans be more fully developed in the beginning phase?" (1964, p. 75). She concludes that social group work theory and practice have not yet given sufficient consideration to the interdependence of worker's individual and group diagnoses and treatment planning and to the means for their synthesis. Thus, Main's research implies that early diagnosis of group members should be incorporated in a model of pregroup planning.

Research by Boer and Lantz (1974) underscores the importance of including factors related to group composition in any model of planning for social work with groups. Research they conducted in which group composition in one group was unplanned and in another planned led them to conclude that "The groundwork of membership selection that occurs before the group has as much importance in determining member commitment, attendance, and therapeutic results as does the ongoing group process" (p. 176).

Social work writing on work with groups, social work research, and social work practice experience all imply that six interrelated and interdependent components would comprise a model of planning for social work with groups. These components are need, purpose, composition, structure, content, and pregroup contact. Thorough and thoughtful pregroup planning would give consideration to the following questions:

–Need. What are the needs of potential group members as perceived by them? by the worker? by the agency? by other relevant persons? What is the need for the group as perceived by potential group members? the worker? the agency? other relevant and/or knowledgeable persons? Can these needs best be met by the group modality?

–Purpose. What are the goals of potential group members as perceived by them? by the worker? What is the tentative conception of the group purpose as viewed by potential members? by the worker? by the agency?

–Composition. How many group members will there be? What will be the characteristics of the group members in regard to sex? age? homogeneity/heterogeneity? educational, occupational, socioeconomic, racial, ethnic, and cultural background? previous group experience? What are the characteristics of a worker who would best work with this group? Will there be one worker or more than one?

–Structure. What will be the duration of each meeting? of the total work? Where will the group meet? How will members get to sessions? What are the resources and supplies that are needed? What is the budget for the group? How will confidentiality be maintained? cooperation and communication with other relevant professionals? Will membership be open or closed?

–Content. What will go on at the meetings? What supplies and/or equipment are needed? How and by whom will content be planned?

–Pregroup Contact. How and by whom will intake, screening, recruitment, and orientation to the group be carried out? What will be the content of intake, screening, recruitment, and orientation processes prior to the first group meeting?

Further work needs to be done in explicating additional components of a pregroup planning model, in discovering the interrelationships among them, and in developing a set of principles to guide the social worker in the actual process of planning.

In 1962, Hartford stated:

> *There is no single comprehensive formulation of group formation process in social science literature. The literature on small group theory and research contains references to group formation and indicates some of the elements of group development, but these are not organized or completely consistent from one author to another. Similarly, there is no clearly formulated or consistent set of principles for group work practice in group formation.* (p. 8)

The gap that Hartford reported 15 years ago remains unfilled today. Development of a planning model that would guide the thinking and preparation of the social worker prior to the first group meeting is needed. Thorough and thoughtful pregroup planning is a necessary prerequisite for group formation that contributes mightily to the success of social work groups. We can ill afford to continue to neglect this important component of practice.

REFERENCES

Bartlett, H. M. Toward clarification and improvement of social work practice: The working definition. *Social Work*, 1958, *3*, 5-8.

Bernstein, S. (Ed.). *Explorations in group work*. Boston: Milford House, Inc., 1973. (a)

Bernstein, S. (Ed.). *Further explorations in group work*. Boston: Milford House, Inc., 1973. (b)

Boehm, W. W. The nature of social work. *Social Work*, 1958, *3*, 10-18.

Boer, A. K., & Lintz, J. E. Adolescent group therapy membership selection. *Clinical Social Work Journal*, 1974, *3*, 172-181.

Briar, S. Family services. In H. S. Maas (Ed.), *Five fields of social service: Reviews of research*. New York: National Association of Social Workers, 1966.

Brody, E. *A social work guide for long term care facilities*. Rockville, MD: National Institute of Mental Health, 1974.

Dewey, J. *Experience and education*. New York: Collier Books, 1938.

Garvin, C. D. *Complementarity of role expectations in groups: Relationship to worker performance and member problem solving*. Unpublished doctoral dissertation, University of Chicago, 1968.

Glasser, P., Sarri, R., & Vinter, R. (Eds.). *Individual change through small groups*. New York: The Free Press, 1974.

Hartford, M. E. *The social group worker and group formation*. Unpublished doctoral dissertation, University of Chicago, 1962.

Hartford, M. E. *Groups in social work*. New York: Columbia University Press, 1971.

Levine, B. *Fundamentals of group treatment*. Chicago: Whitehall Company, 1967.

Main, M. W. *Selected aspects of the beginning phase of social group work*. Unpublished doctoral dissertation, University of Chicago, 1964.

National Association of Social Workers. *Building social work knowledge*. New York: Author, 1964.

Northen, H. *Social work with groups*. New York: Columbia University Press, 1969.

Rosenthal, W. A. Social group work theory. *Social Work*, 1973, *18*, 60-66.

The Significance of Social Group Work Based on Ethical Values

Gisela Konopka

This paper was written and thought through on a day of strong emotions: A folder of extraordinary etchings had arrived in the mail–terrible scenes of experiences in the Nazi concentration camp of Theresienstadt–and a letter accompanying them telling about the artist's deep caring for human beings. They revived not only my own experiences under Nazi persecution but were intermingled with something I had read recently in a newspaper article, a black experience which had apparently touched me so deeply that it had become part of me. The article described a custom at West Point to "freeze out" a person who had done something against the honor code: it is called the "Silence." The cadet has to live in total segregation nobody ever speaks to him. The last paragraph read:

> *The perversion to which this can lead is illustrated by the fact that Lt. Gen. Benjamin O. Davis, Jr., the Air Force's first black general and the son of the Army's first black general, was silenced because of his race for his entire four years (1932-1936) at West Point.* ("Perverting West Point's Honor Code," 1973)

Dr. Konopka is at the University of Minnesota Center for Youth Development and Research, 48 McNeal Hall, 1985 Buford Avenue, St. Paul, MN 55108.

This article was originally published in *Social Work with Groups*, Vol. 1 (2) © 1978 by The Haworth Press, Inc.

[Haworth co-indexing entry note]: "The Significance of Social Group Work Based on Ethical Values." Konopka, Gisela. Co-published simultaneously in *Social Work with Groups* (The Haworth Press, Inc.) Vol. 28, No. 3/4, 2005, pp. 17-28; and: *A Quarter Century of Classics (1978-2004): Capturing the Theory, Practice, and Spirit of Social Work with Groups* (ed: Andrew Malekoff, and Roselle Kurland) The Haworth Press, Inc., 2005, pp. 17-28. Single or multiple copies of this article are available for a fee from The Haworth Document Delivery Service [1-800-HAWORTH, 9:00 a.m. - 5:00 p.m. (EST). E-mail address: docdelivery@haworthpress.com].

What cruelty and horror there is in outcasting a human being. Yet what very rare and almost superhuman capacity of the person who withstood this! How could he have done it? It must have been not only the professional goal he had pursued. He must have been sustained by his inner communication with all his brothers and sisters who suffered too, the same way some of us lived through experiences in isolation cells during the Nazi period. Morris West (1964), the great writer, expressed the terror of utmost isolation of a human being in his book *The Shoes of the Fisherman*. He describes the recurring fear of Kardinal Kiril of being alone, produced by such experience,

> *He had been beaten often, but the bruised tissue had healed itself in time. He had been interrogated till every nerve was screaming and his mind had lapsed into a merciful confusion. From this, too, he had emerged, stronger in faith and in reason, but the horror of solitary confinement would remain with him until he died.* (West, 1964, p. 17)

The human being needs the support of others, as well as to support others. We are physically separate entities but we cannot develop in isolation.

Beyond its significance to the support of individuals, the group is also one of the strongest entities to produce action in human society. Social reformers always knew this. Mary Parker Follett (1934), who came from political science and worked extensively in neighborhood houses and in the field of corrections, wrote:

> *The great cosmic force in the womb of humanity is latent in the group as its creative energy; that it may appear the individual must do his duty every moment. We do not get the whole power of the group unless every individual is given full value, is giving full value.* (p. 39)

She understood that reform movements needed strong groups. The potential of the group process needs to be developed by skilled enablers to achieve active participation by each member. Group work grew out of such understanding of individuals, group process, and society.

I started with the emotional impact of group association on the individual as well as the action-oriented impact of the group on wider movements, because these are the two prongs of social work intent as I understand it. Throughout the history of social work there is questioning of whether it is a profession which serves to just put bandaids on the ills of society by supporting only those who suffer or whether it works to correct the roots of societal evils. The question has frequently been answered with an "either/or." For instance, parts of social work have gone through periods of imitation of psychiatry by intense probing into individual problems. These factions have insisted that this was the only true social work. Other factions want exclusive concern with the "power structure," "management," and consider all other approaches inferior. Clearly any profession whose goal is positive human relations and whose essence is a unique combination of knowledge, skill, and value orientation can be neither exclusively individual oriented nor exclusively general policy oriented. Social work history shows clearly that

> *the answer must be that social work is responsible for attempting both: to help individuals in the framework of existing conditions as well as to help change social institutions.* (Konopka, 1958, p. 194)

I am glad that I used the word *attempt* when I wrote this 20 years ago after intense study of social work history and philosophy. Too many social workers feel guilty for not yet having saved the world from all evil. I sometimes wonder whether it is conceit or masochism that leads them to beat their breasts and constantly decry the shortcomings of their profession.

I have once more to clarify my concept of social work in general before I deal with social work with groups:

–Social work is one of the human relations professions. It is concerned with the wide spectrum of human rights and responsibilities within social relations and social systems.

–It is problem oriented in relation to individuals, groups, institutions, or systems.

–It works within an ethical value system whose premises are the dignity of the individual and mutual responsibility.

–Its practice must take into account understanding of individuals within groups and systems as well as an ethical value system.

Because we recognize more than ever the strength and significance of groups it seems unquestionable that work with groups is one of the central skills of the social worker. Good practice means the unique *combination* of knowledge, philosophy, and method that represents this particular profession. It was from such an integrated vantage point that Grace Coyle in 1940 evaluated the then newly developed T-group approach and discussed it critically in her famous dialogue with Leon

Festinger. (There is no published account of this discussion. Festinger was one of the outstanding followers of Kurt Lewin; they developed "group dynamics" at M.I.T.) She used as a measuring stick for the use of this technique her understanding of individual and group dynamics (knowledge), her ethical concern for "informed consent" of the person, client, or member involved in any social work undertaking (philosophy), and finally her experience of working with groups (method). She neither fell for a new fad nor did she reject the technique because it was new.

In recent years, the flood of novel group approaches to therapy has often caused social workers to adopt the latest fad. I am convinced that each group approach has some important contribution to make–and I will name some of them–but they must be thought through carefully. A professional should not just follow fashion. While group work for too many years was laughed off by social workers, work with groups has become fashionable in a very uncritical way.

The three parameters to consider in determining what practice to use in social work are:

1. Knowledge or at least a good hypothesis regarding the problem to be solved (persons within the system);
2. Ethical philosophy with emphasis on respect for the individual and responsibility of human beings for each other;
3. Skill in translating an enabling attitude into reality.

In the following I will first take a few of the recently fashionable group approaches and discuss them from the point of view of social work as I described it, then bring examples and characteristics of social group work, and finally draw some conclusions about what this means to social work practice in general and the teaching of social work.

T-groups started many years ago under the leadership of Kurt Lewin and his followers (Lewin, Lippit, & White, 1939). They were originally laboratory groups designed to help participants develop an understanding of their own reactions to others, as well as to learn skills in observing group process. The groups were usually quite unstructured and the "trainer" would only enter to facilitate the process when it bogged down. As a learning method for qualified people with no severe emotional problems, this seemed, and still seems to me, an appropriate method. It is a form of learning through doing. Yet this T-group approach soon changed to be used as a global method to help people learn about themselves, in moving them toward optimum performance and interaction with others. "Sensitivity groups" have grown out of this, forcing any participant to do much soul searching.

The problem I see here is that these approaches are often being used indiscriminately without any consideration of (1) how strong a person is to withstand group pressure, and (2) what a negative impact of group pressure can do. People with weak egos can experience serious psychological breakdown or become totally dependent on those group experiences.

The marathon sensitivity groups (Ruitenbeek, 1970, pp. 72-113) which have adopted many of the T-group techniques have added a very serious problem: providing the illusion of warmth and intimacy to people who are deprived of these. They offer "instant" love but seldom provide the inner strength necessary to live through times of solitude or despair. They also allude that "just being open with one another" solves all problems. There is no question that openness in communication is a helpful human tool for learning, but in the reality of the world one must also be aware of times when such openness is inappropriate. One must be especially weary of "pretended" openness or that which is used mainly to hurt or deceive. A helping person should believe in people but be a realist too. In responsible work with people one has to be both. We must know that human beings can be beautiful but they also may want to hurt others. We must not be overly suspicious, yet neither can we be naive and drive others into a world of illusion.

More important, it is one of the tasks of educators and social workers to help people to live in and cope with the real world with strength. Too often, marathon weekends serve as emotional drugs and become a flight from the hard reality in this world (Shaffer & Galinsky, 1974, pp. 148-163). 1 want to be understood: people who consciously choose a way of life that makes weekend sensitivity groups their recreation and marathons their personal outlets have a right to do this–just as others choose mountain climbing or visits to an art museum. But as a social work method, those approaches are neither individualized enough to be responsibly therapeutic nor do they enhance social consciousness, the two social work intents by which any social work method must be evaluated.

Another widespread group approach is based on the theory of *operant conditioning* or *behavior modification* (Skinner, 1953). The theory underlying this is the assumption that the human being learns by success or nonsuccess, or, expressed differently, by reward and punishment. The teacher or social worker who uses operant conditioning is by the nature of this approach placed in a highly authoritarian position. He assumes that he knows what is best for the person. The method is frequently manipulative–it uses reward and punishment to produce a certain kind of behavior, but *without the consent of the group members.*

In social work with people of normal intelligence, this method seems to me unacceptable, though in all of our work we also use some forms of reward–we "support" a person, we give love, recognition, etc. Yet the principle of "informed consent" which grows out of our belief in human dignity does not allow us to manipulate people into what only *we* think is best for them. On the contrary, one of our, and, I might add, education's hardest jobs, is to increase the capacity of people to think for themselves, to learn even to refuse rewards, for instance, if this contradicts their conviction, thinking, concerns. Where would social movements be if people only work for rewards? I know that the answer of the behavior modification theorists is that those people get their inner rewards. Possibly, yes, but where did those rewards come from if all through life comfort and discomfort, success and failure, were the major incentives? There was no glory, no joy, no comfort in fighting the Nazis and dying, tortured and unknown. A democratic society can exist only if citizens get their motivation consciously and clearly from ethical values, not from fear of punishment or expectation of reward.

A second philosophically unacceptable part of behavior modification is the authoritarian position of the individual or group worker. Social group work asks of the group worker that he or she "enable" others to help them become able to make their own decisions. He or she can do this only by interacting with the group members in a process that lets them experience their own thoughts and feelings as well as the thinking and feelings of others.

Behavior modification points with pride to its success with mentally retarded people. It only proves that it is a good "training" method for people with impaired judgment and then only if it is done gently and with more use of reward than punishment. Yet in the case of people who have judgment, it defeats any development of long-range learning to make decisions. It defeats genuine "moral development."

Another group approach claimed as a panacea in work with delinquents is *guided group interaction* (Vorrath & Brendtro, 1974). It is based on the sound assumption that people can learn to help each other and that mutual help is more significant for each member than help by an outsider. This is and has always been a major premise of social group work. But guided group interaction or "positive peer culture" has unfortunately developed into a simplistic technique with specific gimmicks: the group worker, for instance, must sit separate from the group behind a table, or, *all* young people in delinquency institutions *must* join groups. Thus, a sound idea has been distorted because of its routine use and its messianic promises.

Reality therapy (Glasser, 1965) is a countermovement to orthodox psychoanalysis or psychoanalytically influenced casework. It repeats what group work has brought into social work from its early beginnings, namely that help to people comes from looking at the here-and-now as well as at hope for the future. Yet social group work does not entirely reject the significance of the past and will allow a look at it when appropriate.

In this method, the dogmatic singling out of *one* approach alone–that group members are not allowed to talk about the past–distorts an individualized and humane approach to people. Sometimes the past must burst through and be dealt with. This does not mean that the past serves as an "excuse," but even Freud never thought of it that way, nor that it suffices to dwell on the past. Looking at the past may help to work through present problems and to prepare for the future. The assumption, for instance, that one of my young black friends who is preparing for a Ph.D. must never talk about the hurts he lived through while growing up in a Southern ghetto would be cruel and not helpful to him, even though movement comes from his focus on the future.

After having discussed some of the recent group techniques, what then are the most significant characteristics of social group work that make it a sound and central method of social work?

1. The unique integrative view of the individual within the group process and the wider environment (insights derived from psychology, sociology, anthropology, and political science) has preceded the system theory and has proven itself a superb screen of understanding people.

2. The stress of social group work on intellect as well as on feelings, expressed in its use of a wide variety of media such as art, drama, games, and discussions, lends itself to the service of people who are nonverbal as well as verbal. This characteristic proves itself especially significant for work with alienated youth. Also, the school system itself searches for help with an integration of cognitive and affective approaches.

3. The significance of the concept of "member" instead of "client" indicates a democratization of the helping process, an acceptance of the legitimacy of indigenous leadership and the concept of mutual aid as a goal. For instance, relationships between volunteers and professionals are changing. In early social work, the volunteer was "the boss" and the social worker the handmaiden. With professionalization the relation-

ship became reversed and the professional became "boss." Now, with the rise of people in poverty neighborhoods or other repressed groups as significant helpers, an alliance between lay person and professional on an equal basis begins to form.

4. The role of the social group worker cannot be one of a remote authoritarian nor a simple observer nor an echo. All those were roles assumed in times when social work followed the medical model of the all-knowing, benevolent authority. This is past and ineffective today. It is an insult to people, especially to young people, to expect them to open their hearts and souls if the helping person stays remote, is not a person, and is not willing to self-disclose. It does not mean that the group worker should use the group for his or her own therapy. Yet he or she must be a *person* and the group members have a right to know something about him or her. By giving something of oneself, by making the group experience a truly shared one, one can begin to gain the true–not pretended–confidence of people. Then group members can learn to help each other, which is really their need as well as the goal of work with them. They will become free to interact honestly, so that they can learn who they really are from each other. Let me give an example from an institution in which the young people revolted against having groups; the groups had not been forced on them, but the conductor of the group had silently entered each meeting, sat down, and asked them to share their problems.

> The new group worker suggested that the girls should just meet her. When she entered the designated room, only one girl, with curlers in her hair, sitting far away from the seat that was placed for the group worker, was present. The group worker said "hello" and wondered where the others were. The girl said that she wasn't sure whether they would come, but maybe a little later. Then with suspicion she said, "Is this a meeting?" The group worker said that it might be called that, but she was here to think through with the girls what could be done to make this place a more pleasurable and more productive one for everyone who was present. The girl then curled up deeper into her chair and said that she wasn't one to talk. The group worker suggested that that was all right, that she sometimes didn't feel like talking either.
>
> The group worker had been in New Orleans a few days earlier and had brought along some goodies from that city. She gave the box to the girl and suggested she share it with the others. The girl asked what this was, and the group worker said that they were

pralines made by Creoles in New Orleans. The girl picked up on that, and asked what Creoles were. There ensued a lively discussion about Creoles, the city of New Orleans, travel, etc.–all this with a girl who had pronounced that she would not talk at all.

Other girls had been outside of the room, apparently listening, but unwilling to come in. Now they drifted in, one apologizing that she "looked like a mess." The group worker laughed and said that she looked really like a "clean mess," because she had apparently just come out of the shower. The girl nodded. She showed the group worker a necklace with some small tokens from India. The group worker then said that she had traveled in that area, and told a bit about her travels. The girls were all ears. Then they got very interested in the candy. Again there was discussion of why the group worker was traveling to this place, what her job was. All the questions were answered in a simple and direct manner.

At this time, a girl with tears in her eyes came in, saying that she had just heard that her boyfriend might be dying because he had been in an accident. For a moment there was no sound. The group worker put her arm around the girl, said that this was something terrible to live with, and would she want to talk about it? Immediately following this, the other girls also raised questions. The next 15 minutes were filled with a compassionate discussion of the sorrow the girl experienced and the terrifying things one experienced when one got into an accident. One of the girls who lead sat silently, removed from the others, burst out with a "I would just die if my grandmother would die–I couldn't take it because she is the only person who has any meaning in my life!" Another girl said that it was wrong to say that, that somehow one had to live on. A third one said that there was God, and that one could hold onto Him. A fourth one mentioned that she too had felt as if there were no way out anymore when her father died, but after a while she could go on.

She looked at the group worker and asked, somewhat shyly, whether she had ever experienced anything like it. The group worker said that as an older person she certainly had experienced many deaths, but that it was perhaps hardest to take when she was young. She described such an experience. There was warmth in the feeling for each other, and the girls who had said that they would never come to a meeting, that they would not want to have any group sessions in which they discussed anything personal, stayed for approximately 45 minutes.

What is seen here is that the group session means close interaction between the group worker and the youngsters and among the peers themselves. Anything occurring at present is significant to talk about, but it leads into making connections with past and present emotions. There is a warmth of atmosphere that allows the young people to be open with the group worker. The group worker also shares herself.

It is significant to point out that at another session where the same group worker was not present, the girls referred back to their previously discussed concern but enlarged on it and talked about other painful separations.

5. Group content relates to present, past, and future. Group atmosphere needs to be open, warm and accepting. Confrontation should be honest, but also supportive.

Sessions which *force* insight may become phony. Many of our young people are quite sophisticated about the schools of thought which relate emotions and actions to past experiences. They may use group sessions to give lip service to what they think is expected of them, but do not really involve themselves.

Participation, in whatever group and at whatever stage of development of those in the group, is the key word of social group work.

6. Finally, social group work cannot be thought of as a routine technique that can be used under all circumstances in the same way and can be taught through a "cookbook" mechanical approach. It demands a practitioner who has learned to assess people and their situation, knows his or her philosophy, and has the capacity to elicit self-help forces within the individuals and groups. Then, according to their needs and capacities, he or she will develop with the group members various approaches to achieve their goals.

Previously I gave a more explicit example of what may be called a group with therapeutic intent. I would like to describe another example with a community development intent:

> A small group of American Indian women had approached a group worker to help with the following problem: Indian women frequently came from the reservation into the city but were totally unprepared for city life. They did not know how to board buses, how to use telephones and household appliances, did not know social service resources and how to approach them, etc. In discussing the request for help in relation to this, it was agreed that the women would find city-experienced Indian women to meet with the group worker to help them learn how to teach others so that they them-

selves could teach the newcomers. This started a chain of genuine self-help work with leadership emergence within the Indian community.

At this time in history, I cannot perceive of any social service that does not need to include services to groups as well as to individuals and larger units. All social workers should know that all three social work methods–casework, group work, and community organization, as well as newly discovered ones–must be used when needed, and they should be prepared to give them competently. Since the basic knowledge and philosophy underlying all social work practice are the same, it should not be difficult to teach these various approaches in schools of social work and in continuing education to those who learned only one approach in earlier times. The skill is different and can be learned, as we have so successfully developed in social work, in supervised practice. The major learning will occur through reading the literature and working with capable practitioners, but especially by helping students and experienced practitioners to develop their own "art" in working with human beings based on a nondogmatic, flexible, and thought-through philosophy and theory.

Group power has led humanity into the horrors of Nazism and racism; it has made people into conformists and cowards. Group power has sustained those who felt weak and allowed the suppressed to gain dignity. The group is the "atomic" power of human relations. It is important that anyone in human relations and social work be a part of this large field, realize the power of groups, and work toward the betterment of human relations. They must become as Eduard C. Lindeman said many years ago: "something more than a skilled craftsman, something more than a well-meaning idealist" (Lindeman, 1949, p. 221).

REFERENCES

Follett, M. P. *The new state* (4th ed.). New York: Longmans, 1934.

Glasser, W. *Reality therapy.* New York: Harper and Row, 1965.

Konopka, G. *Eduard C Lindeman and social work philosophy.* Minneapolis: University of Minnesota Press, 1958.

Lewin, K., Lippitt, R., & White, R. K. Patterns of aggressive behavior in experimentally created "social climates." *Journal of Social Psychology,* 1939, 10, 271-299.

Lindeman, E. C. *Social work as human relations.* New York: Columbia University Press, 1949.

Perverting West Point's honor code. Minneapolis *Tribune,* June 17, 1973, p. 13A.

Ruitenbeek, H. *The newgroup therapies.* New York: Avon, 1970.

Shaffer, J. B., & Galinsky, M. D. *Models of group therapy and sensitivity training.* Englewood Cliffs, N.J.: Prentice-Hall, 1974.

Skinner, B. F. *Science and human behavior.* New York: The Free Press, 1953.

Vorrath, H., & Brendtro, L. *Positive peer culture.* Chicago: Aldine, 1974.

West, M. L. *The shoes of the fisherman.* New York: Dell Publishing Co., 1964.

The Use of Program:
Review and Update

Ruth R. Middleman

SUMMARY. This paper focuses on what has been thought of in social group work as "program"–program skills, program content, program media, or use of program–and what is now known as nonverbals, exercises, simulations or games, or expressive therapy. Certain dilemmas of the past, e.g., process vs. product (content), talking vs. doing, social work vs. recreation, are reviewed as obstacles to the integration of doing-oriented activities within the major theoretical approaches to group work in social work. Such obstacles have been less encumbering to other professions which have presently assumed the dominant theoretical leadership in this area. Some recent developments in knowledge, technology, and social-cultural forces are described which have contributed to a present milieu that places increased value of diverse modes of expressiveness. The paper concludes with seven future-oriented proposals that theory, practice. and research in this area demand. *[Article copies available for a fee from The Haworth Document Delivery Service: 1-800-HAWORTH. E-mail address: <docdelivery@haworthpress.com> Website: <http://www.HaworthPress.com> © 2005 by The Haworth Press, Inc. All rights reserved.]*

Ruth R. Middleman is Professor, Raymond A. Kent School of Social Work, University of Louisville, Louisville, KY 40292.

This paper was presented at the First Annual Symposium: Social Work with Groups, November 30, 1979, in Cleveland, OH.

This article was originally published in *Social Work with Groups*, Vol. 3 (3) © 1980 by The Haworth Press, Inc.

[Haworth co-indexing entry note]: "The Use of Program: Review and Update." Middleman, Ruth R. Co-published simultaneously in *Social Work with Groups* (The Haworth Press, Inc.) Vol. 28, No. 3/4, 2005, pp. 29-48; and: *A Quarter Century of Classics (1978-2004): Capturing the Theory, Practice, and Spirit of Social Work with Groups* (ed: Andrew Malekoff, and Roselle Kurland) The Haworth Press, Inc., 2005, pp. 29-48. Single or multiple copies of this article are available for a fee from The Haworth Document Delivery Service [1-800-HAWORTH, 9:00 a.m. - 5:00 p.m. (EST). E-mail address: docdelivery@haworthpress.com].

Available online at http://www.haworthpress.com/web/SWG
doi:10.1300/J009v28n03_04

"The use of program" is a concept whose time came and went in so-cial group work's history. It is unknown to social work students today. While it may reside in the nostalgic memories of a few social work edu-cators whose lineage is group work, it has disappeared from the vocabu-lary of the profession. Even those persons once familiar with and perhaps adept in the area (myself included), are now more likely to talk of simulations, gaming, activities, tasks, and role play–not program content, program skills, program media–not the use of program. And yet, more program is used today by more social workers and by more people-workers than ever before. How can this be?

Program is our phoenix. It did not really die despite our neglect. It arises revitalized and soars ever more magnificently today with in-creased prominence and virtuosity. In this paper I aim to review some of the history and forces that may account for this reappearance of our al-most extinct but once familiar, valued phoenix. I shall offer some ideas for its preservation and for the advantage the cultivation and rejoining its flight may bring to the profession. I hope to revive serious consider-ation of that part of group work which dealt with the overt member in-terests that brought participants to group experiences or the content which the worker brought, especially the other-than-talk media of en-gagement.

Currently, this area in group work, traditionally known as program, most likely is known as expressive therapy (music therapy, dance ther-apy, and so forth), or as experiential or whole person learning. Perhaps it is called encounter techniques, exercises, structured experiences, or simply nonverbals. The adjective "nonverbal" has become a noun in its own right: "Let's use a nonverbal." Our students may think the use of expressive media and action-experience was the discovery of Gestalt therapists or growth centers. Family sculpture (or use of tableaux) may seem to be the brain child of family therapists, role play the invention of communication labs or of the behaviorists, while singing, dancing, games, and crafts may appear to be the find of the mental health profes-sionals. Other professions and laypersons have laid claim to these me-dia and use them for their special purposes more than social work. And yet, for group workers, they nag and prod the memory. We have a deja vu: we have been there before!

WHAT IS THIS PROGRAM?

In 1935 Grace Coyle raised the question in the *Survey*, "What Is This Social Group Work?" I ask today, "what is this program?" Program has been a conceptual enigma to our Western way of linear thinking and to our love of dichotomies. First it was the content–an embarrassing, less-than-"professional" content. I tried to show that it was also process (1968) by describing and illustrating through various recorded excerpts, meticulously salvaged over the years, how doing-oriented activities could also be used in addition to discussion to pursue group purposes, e.g., expressing feelings, relating to authority, building social competence, and so forth.

The task of presenting program as process was enormously simplified in those days by two events: (1) Helen Phillips had already described how the social group work method could be used as a process to help group members communicate feelings, use the present reality, and deal with group relations (1957). I merely extended this perspective into the activity realm. (2) Marshall McLuhan aroused the general public to the dilemma of linearity: the medium *was* the message (1964), the process *was* the product–a position more extreme than I ever dared to think.

I was interested in showing program to be *both* content and process. John Dewey had earlier discussed the linguistic necessity that the concepts "building, construction and work" designate both process and product. I added program to this list hoping that program, especially the non-talking "fun and games" seeming content, could find a more respectable place within social group work practice and education. To separate process and product seemed to be a conceptual trap. I used the analogy of the times, "program is a tool," and urged that we think of program more as putty than hammer, i.e., a tool that also changes as it is used (1968:66). I also described program as a "vehicle" through which relationships are made and the needs and interests of the group and its members are fulfilled.

I saw two key values achievable mainly through pursuit of doing-oriented activities: learning the rules of the life-game and learning to innovate, create, and develop one's own unique style of living. Subsequently, I lumped the whole conceptual effort of my 1968 book into two worker skills: *engaging in the medium of the other*, and *proposing a medium presumably congenial to the other* (Middleman & Goldberg, 1974).

A second conceptual trap, which today no longer binds us so harshly, was the dichotomy of talking vs. doing, with doing having some stigma because it looked like the content of recreation, and its use was confined to stigmatized populations, children, and old persons. We now see that there is little value in quibbling over the relative importance of talking and doing as there is merit to the chicken/egg argument. As McLuhan suggested, one need not think that chickens created eggs but can view chickens as the eggs' ingeneous way of producing more eggs. In a similar vein, one can view card games or surgical operation teams or dinner parties as social arrangements with known rules, roles, and processes where what is organized is not the activities but turns at talking. If we adopted Goffman's structural perspective on face-to-face interaction (1964) in order to observe underlying elements of the situations, it is just as valid to view group experience as activities which form the natural home of speech and offer opportunities for talking every now and then.

I now think of program as the content/process that forms the *expressiveness* dimension of group life. The *what* and *how* are inextricably meshed, and are one pole of the process/structure polarity. That is, the process (or function) and the content (the form or idea-to-be-expressed) are in continuous interplay with the structure's demands thus placed upon group experience, for example, who works with whom, and for how long, and so forth. Program structures human interaction. Activities affect what happens at the intrapsychic and interpersonal levels. And the intrapsychic and interpersonal dynamics affect the program. The relationship between program and group relations is reciprocal; neither causes the other.[1]

I now think how mechanical the metaphors *tool* and *vehicle* were–signs of those times! Perhaps today a more organismic analogue would be: program is the group's breath, its expressiveness. It can be used to scream, gasp, scold, exalt, tell, sing, and so forth. Like the sorcerer's apprentice, it can get out of hand and do its own thing. But it is a vital sign, at the core of group life. Although constantly happening, it cannot be taken for granted. Some discipline and control must be exerted over its expression, but as with the human breathing system, we can't restrain it for long without dire consequences.

PROGRAM'S RETURN

A year ago I came upon an article describing the development of a group with reclusive isolates in a Bowery flophouse who had learned to trust no one and talk with no one in order to survive (Brooks, 1978). Initially the worker slipped little notes under the individuals' doors to announce a group meeting. Gradually, they became a group with the worker's imaginative, skillful help. Then there it was: her moving description of a swimming event with crutches left in the corner, with the splashing and talking, and "the stream of mutuality." Every now and then one may still find something about program in the literature.

It was refreshing to note that a recent issue of *Social Work with Groups* (Summer 1979) identified this gap in our literature and focused on returning our attention to groups where a central dynamic was the group's involvement with specific content. Several articles in this issue highlighted group experiences where the central dynamic was the program, e.g., hair dressing to connect with and then work with abused and abusive mothers (Breton, 1979), diary writing for a self/other learning experience (Mackey & O'Brien, 1979), and life change lectures and seminars as a means of offering caring and support to persons suffering stressful life events (Roskin, 1979).

Papell and Rothman (1979:99-100) reflected on the importance of program content and cited three sources that have contributed to renewed interest by group practitioners: (1) the humanistic movement's emphasis upon experiential exercises and simulations to achieve group purposes, (2) the behaviorist movement's focus on concrete, specified activities to produce desired outcomes, and (3) the interest of many in the helping professions in learning and conveying knowledge or content.

Let me extend this useful list. We inhabit a different world today and possess a more flexible world view, partly from a knowledge explosion that can inform our practice, partly from shifts in external socio-political-economic forces. Although one cannot really separate these two influences, I shall start with new knowledge. Here I would include: (1) increased awareness of how individuals deal with the world, (2) sophistication in matters of value diversity and power as determinants of problem definition and social context, and (3) in-depth study of the particulars of professional work. In each of these areas we find new bodies of knowledge to inform group practice.

NEW KNOWLEDGE

We now know more about the diversity of individual functioning and are more tolerant of such differences. The frontiers of knowledge about perception and information processing have been extended. We know there are many roads to Rome despite academia's preference for empiricism and the methods of knowledge acquisition of the physical sciences. Occasionally, questions are raised as to the appropriateness of the analytic scientist's style of inquiry as sufficient for the social sciences and of Aristotelian logic as necessarily preferred in dealing with human systems (e.g., Mitroff & Kilman, 1978). We have information that challenges a U.S.A. egocentrism. The culturally relative patterns of behavior and use of time and space have been described (Hall, 1959), as well as cultural diversity in preferred social philosophies, and even valued thinking patterns. For example, while our tradition emphasizes inductive and pragmatic reasoning, other nations may value intuitional, deductive, or dialectic patterns of thinking (Pribram, 1949). Transpersonal psychologies (Tart, 1975) and Eastern modes of knowing are seen by many as not inferior to the ways of science. We know more about right brain hemisphere functions and a new dignity surrounds the intuitive, holistic, artistic, nonlogical modes of experiencing and knowing (Ornstein, 1972; Watzlawick, 1978). We see the emergence of study of cognitive styles (Messick, 1976). These are pervasive determinants of individual differences in dealing with the world possibly more important for understanding and valuing individual performance than IQ and ability tests, especially for social work's populations of concern. All of these developments affect how practitioners now deal with clients. We value metaphor and analogy, fantasy and imagery, lateral thinking or Po (de Bono, 1972), visual thinking (Arnheim, 1969), nominal groups (Delbecq et al., 1975), brainstorming and other routes to conceptual blockbusting (Adams, 1974), idea production, and creativity. Social workers now have more knowledge to inform and direct our long held value of respect for individual difference.

Problem Definition and Social Context

I shall list only a few among the many areas of knowledge that have extended our concept of problem definition and social context. It is beyond my main focus to deal in depth with our increased sophistication with shifting problem definitions, with the economic-political determinants of programmatic imperatives, with the funding and researchability determinants of social responsiveness and which "experts" may direct the action plans, with the fads and fashions, and with the professional in-fighting when resources become slim. At a less lofty level, so far as present enthusiasm for the use of program is concerned, I identify some key influences.

We find increased concern for health as well as illness and for the expansion of consciousness through diverse resources for expression and self-realization. Some interest and priority is now directed to prevention although still determined more from medical and countable perspectives than public health and social requirements. Theoretical and empirical advances in communication and nonverbal communication have transformed the esoteric into common knowledge, e.g., today's fairly popular idioms of "body language," "personal space," and "dress for success." Theory development in terms of roles, systems, adult development, personality, small groups, and social work practice have led us to evolve group approaches where emotions are directly dealt with, where behaviors are practiced and taught, where interpersonal competence is overtly specified as an organizing goal, and so forth.

Knowledge About Professions and Occupations

The paraprofessional and technician movements have highlighted for all professions the importance of the concrete particulars, of the many services fruitfully rendered by less comprehensively educated service providers, of the impossibility of meeting human needs with a slim, elite group of highly trained professionals. The non-professionals' very concreteness, telling and showing, advising and demonstrating in everyday language has served to highlight the nitty-gritty as appealing, important, and helpful to consumers. Self-help groups, which are said to involve 15 million participants today (Reissman, 1979), are a real challenge that professionals are now trying to get with rather than ignore. Their use of inspiration and member-to-member emphasis cannot be dismissed as valued ways of helping. Worker tasks and job components are now analyzed (Fine & Wiley, 1971) and performances are considered more carefully. The search for competence measures, by the professions, business and government, led to the use of interactional tasks and simulations as potentially fruitful measures of knowledge application and performance. These approaches contrast with paper and pencil tests which are more apt to measure knowledge about or skill in test taking (McClelland, 1973). Such approaches to skills assessment now exert influence in higher education, management assessment centers, and group services. We have become a skills-conscious society that pressures people to develop and keep up their skills; and we are knowledgeable about the training and instructional technology to teach skills.

The group worker now has a rich, even overwhelming, literature to explore to deal with individual and group experience and expressiveness–with consciousness raising, consciousness expanding, and consciousness confronting. There are modules and designs for all kinds of structured experiences to tap the domains of awareness, values, affect, ideas, information, and behavior (e.g., Pfeiffer & Jones, 1972 and on).

EXTERNAL SOCIAL FORCES

While technical information, theory, and research have extended the group practitioners' vistas, the social surround has also changed. I shall list some key influences although they are neither mutually exclusive nor comprehensive: (1) the press toward specialization and diversification, (2) the impact of technology, and (3) shifting values.

Specialization and Diversity

As the average level of formal education rises each year, we find diversification in taste and interests, and many overspecialized workers who suffer boredom in routinized positions and long for outlets for creative energies, imaginative thinking, and self-expression. Bureaucratization has dehumanized and routinized many tasks. Regimentation in education has diverted many from academic or white collar preparation entirely; the rewards are simply not worth the pain of pursuit. We have been warned by Fuller (1975) that overspecialization in biology has led to loss of general adaptability, even extinction of certain life forms. In human terms it has led individuals to lives of desperate isolation and single mindedness.

Technology

Technology has made housework simpler; the women's movement has lent support to many who formerly thought they had to like it. Second careers are more prevalent as well as longer life spans after retirement. There are more hours to be filled in non-work related ways. The workweek grows shorter, the marketplace needs less personpower, and the very importance of work is questioned increasingly by more segments of the population. Increased leisure and affluence stimulate interest in cultural and recreational pursuits, travel, health and athletics, and activities that once seemed esoteric or frivolous. And television brings immediacy and familiarity with diversity and acquisitiveness to all segments of society.

Values

The civil rights and subsequent rights movements have increased tolerance for diversity in life styles, expressiveness, and values to a certain extent. Play is more valued for the young and old alike as a necessary outlet for unused energies. Joyful pursuits are less sinful. There is awareness of and concern for the quality and the qualities of life. Without detailing these value shifts further, we see that our cultural surround has changed. Much that was once the special province of group workers is now commonplace.

THE POPULARIZATION OF GROUP WORK'S DOMAIN

Folk songs no longer are what a few learned at Girl Scout Camp. Arts and crafts appear periodically at public fairs. Do-it-yourself books exist for every imaginable handicraft, from abstract painting to zither-making. Shops for the exotic, the ethnic, the special foods once remote, and all the activities and dances that were specialities of the Settlement House have come to Main Street. Special interest groups, once the mainstay of Ys and centers, abound in most communities now. Mainly, they are self-help affairs and meet all varieties of human need: for the simpler life, the primitive, the small community; for the expression of emotionality and exploration of relationship; for in-group identity support; for stigma reduction, status enhancement, and shared problematic situations (Back & Taylor, 1976). Those who can recall the *U.S. Handbook for Recreation Leaders* can now find our old games as TV fare, computerized games, or commercial board games. Remember Cootie? Battleship? Charades? In the age of the Muppets, who is naive about puppets?

SOME HISTORY

Group workers no longer need to introduce certain pursuits that are now well known to every person. So much the easier for us! But while we had a head start in these matters, we stopped doing our homework. The history of activities within group work and social work reveals a spotty commitment at best. Let us look back.

Probably the earliest group work theorist who accorded centrality to games and play, folk culture, and activity in group approaches was

Neva Boyd. Her emphasis upon prevention and the development of individual potential through group life is now an accessible component of
group work literature (see Simon, 1971), although she was largely ignored for many years and perhaps out of step with mainstream social
group work. In 1919 Boyd wrote of "the curative power of games" with
the World War I wounded veterans at Camp Custer, of the sluggish
wounds that failed to heal after months of ordinary treatment showing
"remarkable improvement through pleasurable exercise and quick-
ened interest in the normal things of life" (1919:4). Gladys Ryland
contributed substantially to serious study of the potentialities of different program media in writing and through her influence as teacher
upon many of us who were her students (Ryland, 1947; Wilson &
Ryland, 1949, Pt. II).

But those persons who used and valued program were regarded more
as Cinderellas than Snow Whites by the emerging profession of social
group work, and as Mad Hatters by the caseworkers. When the early
group workers moved closer to the social work profession, those who
came from the play, recreation, and leisure time programs were viewed
with skepticism. Wilson described "the scorn of other social work practitioners to 'those workers who play with children, run dances, go
camping or teach arts and crafts' and the question raised at the 1936
California Conference of Social Work as to whether group workers
were social workers" (1976:25). A reliable grapevine has it that Edith
Abbott maintained, "there will never be tiddledywinks in Cobb Hall."

Without question, group workers gained much by identifying with
the developing profession of social work when they left the American
Association of Group Workers in favor of the NASW. But there were
losses, largely not remembered or discussed:

Loss 1: The Flight from Activities in Favor of Talk

To fit in, the social group workers played down their involvement
with and knowledge about using activities and the special interests of
group participants as a point of engagement and became, like caseworkers, helpers who talked. I have described the gradual abandonment of
program and media in more detail elsewhere (1968:15-63). By 1959 the
CSWE Curriculum Study of Social Group Work ranked the three educational objectives about program (among 17) at the tail end. Program
was an "unsolved problem." Where should it be learned: in the rest of
the university? through "life-learning" experiences? through individual
initiative? in class? in field? for credit? for whom? all social work stu-

dents? no social work students? (Murphy, 1959:50-52,70,71). This area of group work curriculum was reported as "more uneven" than the other parts. There was "sensitivity about it from faculty, agency staff and students."

All this only 13 little years after Coyle's landmark statements that differentiated group work from recreation (1947a, 1947b) and lodged group work within social work (1947c), a task she began to conceptualize formally in the mid-30s (1935). Coyle spoke of the two dimensions of group work–activities and the interplay of personalities–as creating the group process, and she urged the worker to deal with *both*. "Program and relationships are inextricably intertwined . . . the use of the human relations involved (are) as important as the understanding and use of various types of program" (1947a:202-203). Coyle remained concerned with both parts of group work although, curiously, she referred to program making as an "art" (1949). But mainly, conceptual energies thereafter were devoted to clarifying the social group work method and the relationships part.[2]

The year 1959 also had personal significance aside from the appearance of the Curriculum Study. In that year I presented my first paper at an Annual Program Meeting of the Council on Social Work Education. At the time I was only a part-time Lecturer at the University of Pennsylvania School of Social Work. Helen Phillips invited Dick Lodge and me to join her in a session chaired by Betty Hartford that was devoted to *Methods of Teaching Social Group Work* (1959). Happily, I accepted. My paper dealt with "Teaching the Use of Program in Social Group Work" and represented a first opportunity for this content to be considered by social group work educators. At the time I was blissfully unaware of the findings of the Curriculum Study.

Loss 2: The Move Beyond Members' Interests

In leaving education and recreation behind, group workers also interpreted more vigorously "starting where the person is" to include subtle pursuit of more than the "where." It became important to pursue goals of democratic decision making, intergroup cooperation, and other social, "professional" values along with the group members' overt interests. It was not unusual to find interracial objectives foremost to the worker and basketball winning foremost to the group member. Like casework, group work went through its period of "social working" others without their awareness and/or consent.

Loss 3: Study and Research on Group Process

Group workers also parted company with the early group dynamics movement in favor of an action and service mission, not simply a study and research interest in group processes *qua* process. Newstetter, Coyle, Hearn, and Deutschberger were closely related to other social scientists who remained mainly committed to the study of groups more than individuals' change through group experiences (at least through the mid-1960s). However, social group workers increasingly used groups to help individuals grow and change and adopted new psychological and personality theories to guide their work. Since those times, outside social work, virtually every psychological school of thought conceptualized for understanding the individual has been transported into a group approach, most often with little attention to what the practitioner should do differently because the approach is a *group* one, other than work with individuals, group watching. Present estimates of the numbers of different group approaches range from about 30 to well over 100.

Loss 4: Focus Upon the Group to Meet Common Problems and Needs

The earlier focus upon common problems, situations, and needs also diminished as group workers joined social work, and took their method into "special settings"–the hospitals, guidance clinics, prisons, etc. Instead of a focus on "the group" and its potential and interests, the focus gradually shifted to the individuals in the group. The early group workers saw problems as inhering more in the press of the social situation than in the defects of individuals and devoted energies to the maximization of participants' talents and strengths. They did much showing and telling, and pressuring the politicians for various environmental reforms. Even well into the 1940s the person with "special" emotional or personality problems was served through the peer group or, if this were too disruptive to the group, was referred for individual attention to a casework agency or psychiatric clinic (Wilson, 1941).

SOCIAL GROUP WORK IN SOCIAL WORK

In joining the profession of social work we gained an identity and willingly pursued issues and problems of pressing importance and value, but the cost was great. Social group work was conceptualized and regarded as one of three major methods. But workers who specialized in practicing a social group work approach were never more than a tiny minority in numbers, 6% in the late 1960s with 1% of the work force actually using group interventions as their primary service method (Stamm, 1968) in a profession that turned to psychiatry for its consultation about groups.

Our professional education offered a broad perspective for viewing social problems and interventions. We knew about reaching out, about social context, about supervision and administration, as well as about the doing-oriented activities. And our knowledge and energies were consumed within the larger context: conceptualizing and teaching social group work; community organization; generalist practice; administration and leadership of our national professional organizations, schools of social work, agencies, government programs; training, program development, and so forth. By and large, we did not stick to leading the small group, to submitting group theories to systematized research, to moving beyond description of our concepts, practice principles, and methods.

Understandably, those devoted to the study and utilization of the program component within social group work were the tiniest minority of all. But over the years some literature in this area has been reported (e.g., Middleman, 1954; Gump & Sutton-Smith, 1955; Churchill, 1959; Middleman, 1968; Klein, 1960; Middleman, 1970a, 1970b; Shulman, 1971; Gentry, 1972; Vinter, 1974; Whittaker, 1974; Feldman & Wodarski, 1975; Kolodny, 1976).

For many, knowledge about groups and program media was applied to the class as group as they became social work educators. Some literature developed on exploring media as teaching methodology (e.g., Abels, 1970; Middleman & Goldberg, 1972). In this area, probably the most useful literature was produced by Bertha Reynolds who did not come from group work but crossed the boundaries between group, individual and community, lending conceptual leadership in all areas as well as in a teaching approach that predated experiential teaching/learning in other professions.

Because of the relevance for our consideration of program, let us consider some of the innovations she described (1942). In the area of "Subject Matter in Its Place," she described the dilemma of either letting "subject matter blind the teacher to the active responses of living persons" or, after outliving "the stage of expounding," seeing student talk as more important than any content the teacher might bring. She described how to teach through discussion: how to start off with a little common story or constructed generalized case instance, "the minia-ture." She also described how to lead in-service groups building upon job-related problems, how to rank order ideas and select priorities (something we now call "posting"), how to teach "anything: in a variety of ways," how to listen to the group–but make it more than a rap session, and how by session three, the leader must "show his goods." Reynolds did "laboratory teaching" long before any NTL, and described "drama-tization of interviews" before there was a concept called role play. Her "working notebook" is now thought of as a learning log or diary. Her "projects" and "experiments" on observation and interviewing, and her teaching of recording by means of "headlined paragraphs" illuminated the best of what is now known as discovery or experiential teaching/ learning. Reynolds lamented a teaching that had to appear "dignified and largely routine" and prided herself on using her "life experience as a first condition for learning and information giving . . . and even Mother Goose as a resource!"[3] Many of these innovations are now becoming standard fare in enlightened teaching and training approaches where whole person learning, participatory instruction, and experiencing are valued.

UPDATE

I have returned to some remembrance of things past not to repeat it or urge any return to it. The times have changed, the structure of the pro-fession has changed, and the practice priorities of the profession are greatly expanded. Tropp (1978) has described social group work as al-most vanished within the larger social work; I (1978) have identified solo leadership and practitioner attention to the group process and be-tween-member communication as casualities in many of the group methods used today. My hopes for social work with groups are twofold: (1) that *all* social workers be able to use group approaches as comfort-ably and knowledgeably as individual ones; (2) that specialization, as presently being developed at master's level, in agencies, and by those in private practice, reflect a specialized group knowledge and skill inclu-sive of the *social* orientation that was the special contribution of group workers.

Our earlier focus upon "normals" and their learning, upon wellness, enhancement, and competence, may be returning to professional at-tention, more from outside influences than from social workers–from humanistic psychology, growth centers, psychological education (see

Alschuler, 1973), counseling and guidance (Ivey & Alschuler, 1973), organization development, self-help activitists, through training (Middleman, 1977), and especially through what I have described as structured groups (in press). Perhaps we can redirect more of our energies and those of our colleagues in the profession toward such goals. It is encouraging to note that Henry Maier, who produced a seminal volume on child development (1965), is now writing one on play, that Norma Lang teaches "non-deliberative approaches in social work practice aimed to explore forms of help additional to those based primarily on verbal, deliberative, rational, and linear problem-solving methods,"[4] that publication opportunities await those who would write and conceptualize such areas further.

For the Future

1. It is no longer tenable to develop partial theories of group practice. Theories that deal only with the serious and seemingly rational side of group life, theories that do not account for the deliberate involvement in the expressiveness dimension, in the non-rational, the creative, the affective, the unexpected, and the spontaneous leaps that the group practitioner can expect will occur are incomplete. Considering our U.S. tradition of pragmatism, where such value is placed on what individuals and groups *do*, it would seem that our theory development must more fully account for this reality.

2. We can separate expressiveness from therapy. There is no logical reason why the use of non-talking media should be thought of as therapy, except that psychology and psychiatry have done more conceptual homework than we have or perhaps that social workers are continuing to buy into other professions' service models for political, economic, or prestige gain. The group work of social work should look different from that of psychotherapy; our profession remains concerned about situations as well as persons.

3. The expressive media now inhere in our *zeitgeist* so we probably do not need to teach or introduce learners to what it "feels like" to be involved in diverse group or solitary modes of expression. But we can lend energy to combat what I call a cookbook mentality that threatens to make the content a "thing" again. That is, the very prevalence and popularity of experiential group approaches and the vast literature available on specific techniques and structured experiences have led to a certain mechanization of group leadership approaches. We can contribute to a

more thoughtful, differential use of techniques, one that moves from practice principles to activities rather than vice versa.

4. Since social work now allows for independent and private practice, perhaps more skilled and experienced practitioners will remain in direct group practice. We may be able to study and more systematically examine group practice empirically and develop more discrete knowledge about the impact of various modes of behavior. In the activities realm we might pick up the kind of exploration Vinter and others at Michigan attempted (Vinter, 1974) and that I undertook (1968), and move beyond descriptive accounts of program. We now possess the methodology and technology for in-depth study of behavioral strategies (e.g., Mann, 1972). Advanced study of the use and impact of activities and nonverbal communication are areas deserving further exploration (e.g., Ephross, 1969; Middleman, 1971; Rubeiz, 1972; Goldberg, 1972).

5. We can devote energy to the development of "outsight" (see Jones, 1968), as well as insight. That is, we can push ahead our special know-how within delivery systems, at client and staff levels, about the effects of social confirmation and shared common problems on individual functioning.

6. Currently, much that group work was always about is now called "prevention." Despite the grandiosity of this claim, there is much that skilled, knowledgeable group practitioners can contribute here. I refer to the increased community awareness about the use of the arts in mental health,[5] about networks and self-help groups, about consultation and education. New opportunities for group approaches also need development in the world of work. The imperatives for informed programs, proposals, and service delivery that utilize our know-how are abundant.

7. Finally, we can highlight to the rest of the profession and to ourselves the values of fun and joy, of spontaneity and creativity, of humor and playfulness. Moreno showed long ago that acting out is better than repression (1946), that creative expression is more than sublimation. We can tighten the problem situations, ours and clients', with imaginative thinking, openness to new data, and renewed belief in human ingenuity.

NOTES

1. Dialogue with Paul Ephross has enriched my ideas.

2. Konopka accorded an emphasis upon awareness of "program activities and the interplay of personalities within the group" as vital for the practitioner. However she, as others, did not deal with this area when the components necessary for the knowledge base were enumerated (Konopka, 1963:14-15).

3. Personal correspondence, February 15, 1974.
4. Personnel correspondence, 1979.
5. See *NASW News*, (October 1979).

REFERENCES

Abets, Paul. "Education Media and Their Selection," in Marguerite Pohek (ed.), *Teaching and Learning in Social Work Education*, New York: Council on Social Work Education, 1970, 59-72.

Adams, James L. *Conceptual Blockbusting: A Guide to Better Ideas*, San Francisco: W. H. Freeman, 1974.

Alschuler, Alfred S. *Developing Achievement Motivation in Adolescents*, Englewood Cliffs, NJ: Educational Technology Publications, 1973.

Arnheim, Rudolf. *Visual Thinking*, Berkeley: University of California Press, 1969.

Back, Kurt and Rebecca C. Taylor. "Self-Help Groups: Tool or Symbol?" *Journal of Applied Behavioral Science* 12 (July-August-September), 1976.

Boyd, Neva L. *Hospital and Bedside Games*, Chicago: Boyd, 1919.

Breton, Margot. "Nurturing Abused and Abusive Mothers: The Hairdressing Group," *Social Work With Groups* 2 (Summer), 1979, 161-174.

Brooks, Ann. "Group Work on the 'Bowery,'" *Social Work with Groups* 1 (Spring), 1978, 53-63.

Churchill, Sallie R. "Prestructuring Group Content," *Social Work* 4 (July), 1959, 52-59.

Coyle, Grace L. "What Is This Social Group Work?" *Survey*, May 1935.

Coyle, Grace L. "Group Work as a Method in Recreation," *The Group* 9, (April), 1947a; and "Social Group Work in Recreation," *Proceedings of the National Conference of Social Work, 1946*, New York: Columbia University Press, 1947b.

Coyle, Grace L. "On Becoming Professional," *Toward Professional Standards*, New York: American Association of Group Workers, 1947c.

Coyle, Grace L. "The Art of Program-Making," *Group Work with American Youth*, New York: Harpers, 1949.

deBono, Edward. *Po: A Device of Successful Thinking*, New York: Simon & Schuster, 1972.

Delbecq, Andre L., Andrew H. Van de Ven, and David H. Gustafson. *Group Techniques for Program Planning: A Guide to Nominal Group and Delphi Process*, Chicago: Scott Foresman, 1975.

Ephross, Paul. "Social Group Workers' Opinions Regarding the Use of Program Media." Unpublished doctoral dissertation: University of Chicago, 1969.

Feldman, Ronald and John Wodarski. "Programming," *Contemporary Approaches to Group Treatment*, San Francisco: Jossey-Bass, 1975, 80-88.

Fine, Sidney A. and Wretha W. Wiley. *An Introduction to Functional Job Analysis*. Kalamazoo, MI: The Upjohn Institute, 1971.

Fuller, R. Buckminster. "The Wellspring of Reality," *Synergetics*, New York: Macmillan, 1975, xxv-xxxii.

Gentry, Martha E. "Social Simulation Games: Implications for Practice and Education," *Social Work Education Reporter* (May/June), 1972.

Goffman, Erving. "The Neglected Situation," *American Anthropologist* 66, 1964, 133-136.

Goldberg, Gate. "Effects of Nonverbal Teacher Behavior on Student Performance," Unpublished doctoral dissertation: Temple University, 1972.

Gump, Paul and Brian Sutton-Smith. "The 'It' Role in Children's Games," *The Group* 19, 1955.

Hall, Edward T. *The Silent Language*, New York: Doubleday, 1959.

Ivey, Allen E. and Alfred S. Alschuler. "An Introduction to the Field" (of Psychological Education) and other articles of this volume, *Personnel and Guidance Journal* 51 (May), 1973, 591-691.

Jones, Richard M. *Fantasy and Feeling in Education*, New York: New York University Press, 1968, 55-86.

Klein, Alan F. "Program Utilization in Social Group Work," redated (circa 1960).

Kolodny, Ralph. "Treatment Considerations in the Use of Program Activities," *Peer-oriented Group Work for the Physically Handicapped Child*, Boston: Charles River Books, 1976, 74-150.

Konopka, Gisela. *Social Group Work: A Helping Process*, Englewood Cliffs, NJ: Prentice-Hall, 1963.

Mackey, Richard A. and Bernard A. O'Brien. "The Use of Diaries with Experiential Groups," *Social Work With Groups* 2 (Summer), 1979, 175-180.

Maier, Henry. *Three Theories of Child Development*, New York: Harper & Row, 1965.

Mann, John. *Learning to Be: The Education of Human Potential*. New York: Free Press, 1972.

McClelland, David C. "Testing for Competence Rather than Intelligence," *American Psychologist* 20 (January), 1973, 1-14.

McLuhan, Marshall. *Understanding Media: The Extensions of Man*, New York: McGraw-Hill, 1964.

Messick, Samuel A. and Associates. *Individuality in Learning*. San Francisco: Jossey-Bass, 1976.

Middleman, Ruth R. "Arts and Crafts as a Group Centered Program," *The Group* 18, 1954.

Middleman, Ruth R. *The Non-Verbal Method in Working with Groups*, New York: Association Press, 1968 (republished, Practitioners Press, Hebron, Conn., 1980).

Middleman. Ruth R. "Engagement Through a Nonverbal Approach," *Voices: The Art and Science of Psychotherapy* 6 (Spring), 1970a.

Middleman, Ruth R. "Let There Be Games," *Social Service Review* 4a (March), 1970b.

Middleman, Ruth R. "The Impact of Nonverbal Communication of Affect on Children from Two Different Racial and Socio-Economic Backgrounds," unpublished doctoral dissertation: Temple University, 1971.

Middleman, Ruth R. "A Teaching/Training Specialization Within the Masters Curriculum," unpublished paper, Council on Social Work Education, Annual Program Meeting, 1977.

Middleman, Ruth R. "Returning Group Process to Group Work," *Social Work with Groups* 1 (Spring), 1978, 15-26.

Middleman, Ruth R. "The Pursuit of Competence through Involvement in Structured Groups," in Anthony N. Maluccio (ed.), *Building Competence in Clients*. New York: The Free Press, in press.

Middleman, Ruth R. and Gale Goldberg. "The Interactional Way of Presenting Generic Social Work Concepts," *Journal of Education for Social Work* 8 (Spring), 1972, 48-57.

Middleman. Ruth R. and Gale Goldberg. *Social Service Delivery: A Structural Approach to Social Work Practice*, New York: Columbia University Press, 1974.

Mitroff, Ian I. and Ralph H. Kilmann. *Methodological Approaches to Social Science*, San Francisco: Jossey-Bass, 1978.

Moreno, Jacob L. *Psychodrama*, Beacon, NY: Beacon House, 1946.

Murphy, Marjorie. *The Social Group Work Method in Social Work Education: A Project Report of the Curriculum Study, XI*, New York: Council on Social Work Education, 1959.

NASW News. "Murky Picture for Arts in Mental Health Programs," 24 (October), 1979, 11.

Ornstein. Robert E. *The Psychology of Consciousness*, San Francisco: Freeman, 1972.

Papell, Catherine P. and Beulah Rothman. "Editorial," *Social Work with Groups* 2 (Summer), 1979, 99-100.

Pfeiffer, J. William and John E. Jones. *Annual Handbook for Group Facilitators*, 1972 on; and *Structured Experiences for Human Relations Training*, Vol. 1 on, 1969-: University Associates, San Diego.

Phillips, Helen U. *Essentials of Social Group Work Skill*, New York: Association Press, 1957; republished, University of Pennsylvania School of Social Work and Norwood. 1973.

Pribram, Karl. *Conflicting Patterns of Thought*, Washington, D.C.: Public Affairs Press, 1949.

Reissman, Frank. "Self-Help: A Strategy for the New Professional Movement?" *The New Professional* 1 (May/June), 1979.

Reynolds, Bertha C. *Learning and Teaching in the Practice of Social Work*, New York: Faraar & Rhinehard, 1942 (Republished, 1972).

Roskin, Michael. "Life Change and Social Work Group Intervention," *Social Work with Groups* 2 (Summer), 1979, 117-128.

Rubeiz, Ghassan M. "Program Content in Group Work: An Empirical Analysis," unpublished doctoral dissertation: Washington University, St. Louis, 1972.

Ryland, Gladys. "The Place, Use and Direction of Program Activities," *Toward Professional Standards, AAGW*, 1945-6, New York: Association Press, 1947.

Shulman, Lawrence. "'Program' in Group Work," in *The Practice of Group Work*, William Schwartz and Serapio Zalba, eds., New York: Columbia University Press, 1971.

Simon, Paul (ed.). *Play and Game Theory in Group Work: A Collection of Papers by Neva Leona Boyd*, Chicago: University of Illinois at Chicago Circle, 1971.

Stamm, Alfred M. "NASW Membership: Characteristics, Deployment, and Salaries," *Personnel Information* 11 (March), 1968.

Tart, Charles T. (ed.). *Transpersonal Psychologies*, New York: Harper & Row, 1975.

Trecker, Harleigh. "The Program Development Process," *Social Group Work*, New York: Association Press, 1972, 102-119.

Tropp, Emanuel. "Whatever Happened to Group Work," *Social Work with Groups* 1 (Spring), 1978, 84-94.

Vinter, Robert. "Program Activities: An Analysis of Their Effects on Participant Behavior," in Paul Glasser, Rosemary Sarri and Robert Vinter (eds.), *Individual Change Through Small Groups*. New York: Free Press, 1974, 244-257.

Watzlawick, Paul. *The Language of Change*, New York: Basic Books, 1978.

Whittaker, James K. "Program Activities: Their Selection and Use in a Therapeutic Milieu," in Paul Glasser et al., *ibid.*, 233-43.

Wilson, Gertrude. *Group Work and Case Work: Their Relationship*, New York: Family Welfare Association of America, 1941.

Wilson, Gertrude. "From Practice to Theory: A Personalized History," in Robert W. Roberts and Helen Northen (eds.), *Theories of Social Work with Groups*, New York: Columbia University Press, 1976, 1-44.

Wilson, Gertrude and Gladys Ryland. *Social Group Work Practice*, Pt. II, Boston: Houghton Mifflin, 1949.

Meeting Practice Needs:
Conceptualizing the Open-Ended Group

Janice H. Schopler
Maeda J. Galinsky

Open-ended groups are an important part of the everyday practice of social workers. In many settings, clients join groups in progress and attend as many sessions as their needs warrant. Professionals lead open-ended groups in general and psychiatric hospitals, social services departments, mental health centers and family service agencies, drug and alcohol rehabilitation centers, residential treatment facilities, nursing and maternity homes, and prisons. Further, many self-help endeavors such as Alcoholics Anonymous, Parents Anonymous, and Recovery, Inc. take place in open-ended groups. The professional literature and conversations with practitioners attest to the number and variety of open-ended groups.[1] Patterns of implementation and attendance vary from waiting-room groups with almost a complete turnover every session to groups that endure for years with occasional revisions in composition. The important theme of changing membership does, however, serve to link these groups together conceptually.

Janice H. Schopler, ACSW, is Assistant Professor and Maeda J. Galinsky, PhD, is Professor, School of Social Work, University of North Carolina, 223 East Franklin Street 150 A, Chapel Hill, NC 27514.

This paper was presented at the NASW 7th Biennial Professional Symposium, Philadelphia, Pennsylvania, November 18-21, 1981.

This article was originally published in *Social Work with Groups*, Vol. 7 (2) © 1984 by The Haworth Press, Inc.

[Haworth co-indexing entry note]: "Meeting Practice Needs: Conceptualizing the Open-Ended Group." Schopler, Janice H., and Maeda J. Galinsky. Co-published simultaneously in *Social Work with Groups* (The Haworth Press, Inc.) Vol. 28, No. 3/4, 2005, pp. 49-68; and: *A Quarter Century of Classics (1978-2004): Capturing the Theory, Practice, and Spirit of Social Work with Groups* (ed: Andrew Malekoff, and Roselle Kurland) The Haworth Press, Inc., 2005, pp. 49-68. Single or multiple copies of this article are available for a fee from The Haworth Document Delivery Service [1-800-HAWORTH, 9:00 a.m. - 5:00 p.m. (EST). E-mail address: docdelivery@haworthpress.com].

Available online at http://www.haworthpress.com/web/SWG
doi:10.1300/J009v28n03_05

Unfortunately, despite the extensive and effective use of open-ended groups there has been little attempt to refine this approach. Theoretical writings pertaining to groups tend to ignore open-ended characteristics and focus on the relatively long-term group with a stable membership. Only scattered attempts have been made to conceptualize the differences in the development of open-ended groups[2] and to denote implications for intervention.[3] Not only are there few guidelines for work with open-ended groups, but lower status has frequently been accorded to groups with changing membership. Practitioners meeting the often overwhelming needs of their clients may apologize to other staff and educators for not working with "real groups." Without recognition or guidelines to direct their efforts, social workers dealing with open-ended groups can find their work frustrating and fraught with unnecessary difficulty.

Our review of the descriptive and theoretical literature related to open-ended groups and our consultation with practitioners provide the basis for this framework for services to open-ended groups.[4] We discuss the purposes for which open-ended groups are appropriate as well as the special considerations that need to be given to composition and group arrangements. Then, we examine the group development, structure, and processes typical of open-ended groups and suggest guidelines for responding to the particular needs of groups with changing membership.

PURPOSES OF OPEN-ENDED GROUPS

Agencies provide services through open-ended groups for a variety of reasons. Open group systems ensure the immediate availability of services, particularly to people in crisis. Clients can begin treatment promptly, obtain information, or be screened to determine what response is most appropriate to their needs.[5] When ongoing support or therapy is required, members can remain in the group as long as necessary and departing members can be offered the option of returning if the need arises.[6] The provision of an open group experience can also be a practical and efficient way of providing support and maintaining chronic patients who return to clinics on a routine basis for medication.[7] In addition, agencies have found open-ended groups in walk-in clinics useful in outreach efforts to provide therapy to deprived clients.[8] Further, agencies committed to training find that ongoing, open-ended client and supervisory groups can offer valuable learning experiences without detriment to clients. The introduction of new facilitators in a client group appears to be no more disruptive than the on-going change in membership;[9] and, supervisory or training groups easily accommodate to the turnover of staff and students.[10] Thus, agencies have developed open-ended groups as a way of becoming more responsive in both service delivery to clients and staff training.

The specific purposes identified in open-ended groups can be categorized as: (1) helping clients cope with transitions and crises; (2) providing other types of short- and long-term therapy; (3) offering support to clients with common problems; (4) assessing or screening clients; (5) orienting and educating clients; (6) training and supervising staff and students; and, (7) facilitating outreach efforts.[11] In some cases, groups appear to have a single purpose such as responding to severely depressed clients to prevent suicide[12] or helping cardiac patients deal with fears of death.[13] In other open-ended groups, multiple purposes are addressed. For example, a group for residents of a maternity home provided education and support as well as an opportunity for client assessment.[14]

Reports from the literature and practitioners indicate that the dominant purpose pursued in open-ended groups is helping clients cope with transitions and crises.[15] Through the open group system, mutual assistance and support are made available to clients who share similar life stresses resulting from: (1) a change in status, (2) change in physical condition, (3) a change in the family system, or (4) a change in the life cycle. Open-ended groups focusing on status changes ease entry into hospitals and nursing homes as well as prepare members for leaving prisons, psychiatric facilities, and residential treatment centers. Open groups dealing with changed physical conditions are offered to patients with cancer, progressive blindness, emphysema, burns, kidney disease, rheumatoid arthritis, as well as recent surgery and stroke patients. Family members meet in open-ended groups to obtain help in coping with stresses related to the birth of a normal or handicapped child, the illness, addiction, or emotional disturbance of a relative, as well as the hospitalization or death of a loved one. Further, open-ended groups are used to help both adolescents and the elderly in dealing with developmental crises.[16]

Groups formed to deal with particular transitions or crises not only offer members the opportunity to exchange perspectives and obtain information in a responsive, nurturing atmosphere but also stimulate problem-solving and the development of coping behaviors. Members experience relief when they know others share their problem. Expressing pent-up feelings, that may be related to the burden of a sick child or the embarrassment of a spouse's addiction, reduces member tensions. Exchanging information provides members with new strategies for dealing with problems such as adjusting to retirement or becoming a parent. As a result of this sharing experience, members feel more confident and able to confront their stressful situations.[17] Further, as members come and go, the group provides a model for dealing with transitions that can enhance each member's capacity for responding to external stress.[18]

While the most frequently mentioned purposes relate to coping with transitions and crises, many open-ended groups are designed for therapeutic purposes, support, and/or screening and orientation. Therapy may involve a psychotherapeutic examination of the past[19] or refer to a more present-oriented problem-solving approach.[20] For psychotherapy groups, changing membership is at times disruptive; and, the only negative description of an open-ended group experience involves traditional group psychotherapy.[21] Support is seldom the sole purpose indicated for a group and is more frequently listed in conjunction with coping with transitions and crises, screening, or therapy.[22] Some groups are designed primarily to assess clients or prepare them for therapy,[23] but screening groups also provide orientation and function as support systems,[24] and, at times, help clients resolve their problems.[25] Although client education or orientation[26] and staff training[27] are rarely mentioned as the main purpose of an open-ended group, it is apparent from the descriptions of these groups that clients are frequently provided with information and learn coping skills; and, that students from a variety of disciplines facilitate open-ended groups as a part of their training experience.

Open-ended groups currently are serving a range of purposes and seem to be a particularly appropriate response to people facing common life crises and transitions. Although the purposes of open-ended groups appear similar to those of groups with stable membership, the leadership demands are different. Knowledge and skills related to group composition and group arrangements in a closed group are not sufficient to deal with the ever-changing membership of an open group.

OPEN-ENDED COMPOSITION AND GROUP ARRANGEMENTS

One of the perennial frustrations of working with open-ended groups is the uncertainty about how many members will attend any given session. Based on reports of open-ended groups, workers can typically anticipate about five to twelve members at a meeting. Workers need to be prepared, however, for as few as one or two members and as many as twenty.[28] Because there is no way to predetermine the actual composition of the group at any session, it becomes particularly important to have a sufficient pool of potential members; this increases the likelihood that enough members will be present at each session for group interaction.

Criteria for group composition are seldom discussed in the open-ended group literature, but self-selection appears to be the predominant mode of composition. The membership pool is defined by the purpose established for the group and individuals who are facing the crisis or problem expressed by the purpose are eligible to join the group. Many groups are completely voluntary and there seems to be an implicit assumption that if the group meets a need, potential members will come. Relatives of burn patients, for instance, are informed about a support group and it is expected they will attend if they are feeling a need to express their concerns or obtain information. Some groups, however, particularly those established for certain categories of clients in treatment centers or in-patient facilities, appear to be less voluntary. An adolescent entering a residential facility or a patient on a psychiatric ward would seem to have minimal choice about joining a group provided as part of the "prescribed" treatment program.

Since potential members may feel some pressure to become part of a designated open-ended group, either because of institutional directives or their physical presence in the meeting area (e.g., ward or waiting room), it is necessary to consider exclusion criteria. Although the purpose may clearly define the population for whom the open-ended group is available, people who are negative about becoming involved, particularly in a therapeutic endeavor, and those who are denying their problems should not be encouraged to attend. If these individuals have pressing needs, they should be addressed through alternative means, such as individual contacts. Attending sessions may induce undue anxiety or resentment and the presence of resistant or unwilling members may detract from the group's work.[29] Care must be taken, however, in excluding members since there are beneficial results from bringing together people with mutual concerns about impending crises or transitions. As with self-help groups, members dealing with a common experience become peers and differences in socio-economic status, education, and occupation often seem unimportant.[30] Facing the death of a child or dealing with the aftermath of surgery can be important common denominators.

People become members of open-ended groups for varying lengths of time. Some groups, such as an aftercare group designed to ease the transition from hospital to community, are available as long as members feel they have a need or reason to come.[31] In other groups, situational factors may determine attendance. An open-ended group on a psychiatric ward had constant turnover because of patient discharge;[32] and, a waiting-room group involved relatives only for the duration of their family member's stay.[33] Further, there may be variable expectations about the number of sessions members should attend. In an open-ended screening group at a community mental health center, members were asked to attend three to six sessions,[34] while a psychiatric walk-in clinic offered ten sessions in an open-ended group to clients coming for short-term treatment.[35]

These examples from the literature emphasize the unpredictable character of attendance in open-ended groups. Although the general presumption is that members attend as long as they find the experience useful, there are no data on why members terminate from open-ended groups.[36] They may leave the group because their needs are met, because they are no longer affiliated with an institution, because they have attended the prescribed number of sessions, or because they do not find the experience helpful.

Changing membership is a dominant force in open-ended groups and practitioners must be prepared to cope with the arrival and departure of members. Members may come and go continually or infrequently but the change in composition is often unplanned. The consequence of changing membership at different points in time is, however, only vaguely defined in the literature and not all of the accounts are in complete accord. Despite the inadequate conceptualization, there are some helpful descriptions of techniques which can ease the impact of change.

Paradise, assuming that open-ended groups progress through defined stages of development, examines the meaning of bringing new members into an ongoing group at different stages. He suggests that any member who enters the group during the first "Pre-Affiliation" stage makes little difference since the group is still forming. During the second "Power and Control" stage, he assumes that a new member is likely to cause frustration and regression since members' relations are tenuous and filled with conflict; thus, it is more appropriate to delay increases in membership until the end of this phase or some point during the third "Intimacy" stage when members may again join with relative ease. Paradise warns that members added during the fourth "Differentiation" stage may be overwhelmed because the group is cohesive and has a defined structure, but indicates the group can incorporate newcomers during this time. In the fifth and final stage of "Separation," he predicts that new members will be poorly accepted since the group is dealing with ending; thus, any change is contra-indicated.[37]

Although there is no research regarding the impact of new members on group development, the literature does provide two descriptive accounts of member entry at different points in time. Duke et al. use Paradise's formulation to discuss movement of an open-ended self-help group through the stages of Pre-Affiliation, Power and Control, Intimacy, Differentiation, and Separation. They conclude that their observations of membership change affirm Paradise's predictions to some extent.[38] Another illustration is given by Scher, who reported on an open-ended aftercare group which met for a ten-year period. He observed that the group took six weeks to adjust to a new therapist or a new member no matter what phase of development members had reached when composition changed. He further noted that members who were in the "middle phase" of their group experience (which might correspond to Paradise's stage of "Differentiation") were the most resentful of any changes.[39]

Ziller's conceptualization is probably the most helpful approach to understanding the phenomenon of changing membership. He proposes that the components involved in assimilating a new member must be examined. These include the characteristics of the newcomer, the characteristics of the group at time of entry, the interaction of these characteristics, as well as the basis for changing membership and the orientation procedures used.[40] Thus, a highly motivated new member with positive group associations whose entry into a receptive group is planned and handled through established orientation procedures should receive a better response than a resident newcomer who arrives unannounced in a group with no mechanisms for assimilating members.

Although Ziller's formulation has not been formally tested, other authors support the need for maintaining a core group or nucleus of members to pass on group traditions and assist in the assimilation of new members;[41] and, a number of authors make suggestions for helping groups deal with membership alterations. When possible, it is recommended that membership changes be paced at regular intervals, rather than adding members at every meeting.[42] Individual group members can share responsibility for "sponsoring" new members and introducing them to the group, a mode used in some self-help groups;[43] and, departing members can be given the opportunity to return if they feel the need.[44] Further, a restatement of the group's purpose and transition exercises for welcoming newcomers and terminating with members who are leaving can lessen the disruption of changing members.[45]

Since practitioners often have little control over who comes to an open-ended group or how long members will attend, it is imperative to define and communicate the purpose of the group to potential members and to determine, in advance, expectations for members and procedures for handling membership change. Further, it is necessary to make arrangements for a meeting place that will be easily accessible and conducive to interpersonal exchange. If the only convenient location is in an open area such as a waiting room, then care must be taken so that the group does not invade the privacy of people who do not wish to attend. To ensure support for group efforts, others who may have contact with potential clients, such as medical personnel and relatives, should be involved. Attending to compositional differences and making appropriate group arrangements lay the groundwork for an effective open group system, but facilitating growth of an open-ended group also requires knowledge of the factors impacting on its development.

OPEN-ENDED GROUP DEVELOPMENT, STRUCTURE, AND PROCESS

There is some question about whether groups with transient members move beyond the initial phases of group development.[46] Certainly, given the great disparity in patterns of attendance, there is ample justification for practitioners' concerns that some open-ended groups never move beyond formative issues. There is, however, substantial evidence that these groups progress and change, even though the changing membership in open-ended groups affects the character of development.

In the open group system, despite the constant turnover in membership, the group itself makes gains over time. There are reports of increased intimacy and interaction. Cohesion develops and members have less need for direction, more ability to make self-disclosures and provide mutual assistance.[47] In Hill and Groner's comparison of the verbal interaction in the development of open and closed groups, there were apparent differences, but a clear indication of movement in open-ended groups when a nucleus from the previous group was maintained. They observed that ongoing open groups made developmental changes (both gains and losses) during periods of stable membership; each time membership changed, however, there was a "continuation effect" so that the newly composed group maintained a developmental level near or slightly lower than the level attained prior to membership change. They concluded that any open group that continued for a long enough period might approximate all the stages of normal development.[48]

It would appear that group development in open group systems, under favorable conditions, goes through a cyclic progression. Depending on how much membership changes and on the stability of the previous grouping, the new group may start from the base established by former members. Within this cycle, Scher points out that individual members vary in their identification with the group and its process. In his observations, newcomers were caught up in becoming part of the group; members already engaged carried on the work of the group; and, terminators began to withdraw.[49] From Scher's portrayal of individual differences in attachment to the group, it might be assumed that a core of engaged members may promote stability and development while a preponderance of incoming and/or outgoing members may slow development.

Ziller discusses the members' time perspective, the group's need for equilibrium, and the frame of reference as factors which can offset the disruptive effects of changing group membership and push group development forward. Because the focus is on the present in open-ended groups, members reach group decisions with greater haste and form attachments to the group, not individuals. Procedures are developed to minimize disequilibrium induced by membership change so the group's work can continue; and, the group profits from the constant reminders of reality and the broader frame of reference offered by new members.[50]

Obviously, not all open-ended groups benefit from the transient nature of their membership. Some find development impeded because of a lack of openness[51] and others are overwhelmed at times by the constant influx of new members.[52] Nonetheless, most of the descriptive accounts of open-ended groups in the literature affirm developmental progress. The mechanisms these groups develop to survive and grow stem from what Ziller might describe as the "group's need for equilibrium." The group's purposes are kept alive by defining goals for newcomers and evaluating departing members' progress.[53] Norms maintain the structure of the group through transitions as established members model and communicate behavioral expectations to new members.[54] In addition to the group factors that aid growth, the development of groups with changing membership can be promoted by a supportive milieu[55] as well as member contacts outside group sessions.[56] Further, leadership, always a critical factor in group progress, is especially important in open group systems. The centrality of the leader is greater than in closed group systems because the leader can carry forward group traditions, provide the structure and information necessary for decision-making, and is often the only constant in the ebb and flow of members.[57]

Over time, open-ended groups may replicate the stages of development that occur in long-term, closed group systems, but they do not move through the stages in an orderly progression. These groups evolve a structure for dealing with changing membership through intermittent and repetitive stages of growth, assimilation, and stabilization. Within open systems individual members or subgroups within the group system can represent different stages of group development; thus, issues related to formation and termination may surface even as the group is dealing with concerns related to the middle phases. For this reason, group development frameworks which stress the repetitive and cyclical nature of groups are particularly useful. For example, Schwartz's framework for group development (tuning-in, beginnings, work, transitions) points to significant phases that occur within a single session as well as the overall process of group development.[58] Sarri and Galinsky's presentation of group development further conveys the cyclic nature of group growth and, if their intermediate and revision stages are repeated continuously, can encompass a substantial part of the pattern of development of open-ended groups.[59]

Practitioners dealing with open-ended groups would be advised to keep in mind both the overall development of the group and the individual progression of members. Every session involves preparation or "tuning in" to the particular demands of change. New members may need to be introduced or departing members may need to deal with separation; and, the work of the group must go on. Since change may be an almost constant phenomenon, the leader must help the group establish mechanisms for dealing with turnover, adapt a leadership style appropriate to the group's development, and create a supportive environment.

Intervention Guidelines for Open-Ended Groups

The practice wisdom derived from this review of the literature on open-ended groups points to the importance of the leader, the group, and the environment. For effective outcomes, it must be recognized that the development of open-ended groups is often dominated by the transient nature of their membership. Leadership skill, a strong group tradition, and a supportive milieu are needed to transform an open group system in a continuous state of flux into a productive, problem-solving network.

Leadership demands. The leader(s) must be prepared for an ever-changing membership, must be attuned to multiple developmental needs within a single session, must be able to define relevant purposes and establish meaningful expectations for members that encompass procedures for dealing with transient membership, and must be able to develop a supportive environment for the group system. Any leader who can meet these demands must have skill in rapid individual and group assessment as well as a leadership style that is adaptive to changing conditions. At any point in the group's development, the leader must have the ability to move into a central position to support group purposes, to activate group traditions, or to ensure the effective operation of mechanisms for dealing with transition. Further, the leader must be able to play a less active, facilitative role if the group is able to manage its own activities.

Group demands. While open-ended groups can be sustained through formative phases with professional guidance, they cannot be expected to progress beyond this phase unless they develop a strong tradition which includes a sense of purpose, expectations for members' behavior, and mechanisms to respond to change Members can ensure that the group's legacy is passed on, and it is especially helpful if a core of members is maintained when old members depart and new members enter. When the group's memory fails, the worker must prompt members to engage in rituals related to welcoming newcomers and evaluating the progress of members who are terminating. Through these exercises, the group reaffirms and clarifies its purposes and expectations.

Environmental demands. A supportive milieu is necessary to an open-ended group system. Membership depends on consistent referrals and reinforcement for participation. Related staff must comprehend the group purpose and their own relationship to the group, if they are to make referrals and promote the group's potential. Members' friends and relatives may need to be alerted to the group's importance if they are to encourage member involvement in the group. Cooperation of significant people in the group's environment can ensure that members attend and benefit from the experience. Even facilitative room arrangements and scheduling may depend on the agency's approval and understanding of the group. Workers need to be sensitive to agency policy and prepared to adjust their plans while advocating for the needs of the group. The smooth operation of an open-ended group and its positive effects on members require supportive relationships.

CONCLUSION

Open-ended groups are an important part of social work technology. There is a dynamic quality about the open group system which is an asset in providing services to clients. In an era of societal stress, open-ended groups provide a mutual aid system which is adaptive to changing membership demands. They serve a variety of purposes and seem especially suited to helping members deal with transitions and crises. Leading a group with changing membership requires an understanding of the multifaceted, cyclic progression of open group systems. Practitioners who hope to obtain successful outcomes must have the ability to assess and adapt to divergent individual and group needs, must be comfortable with a central role in structuring expectations for members and for the group, and must aggressively work to develop a supportive milieu. Transient membership poses a challenge, but the spontaneous relief and creative solutions produced in the interaction of open group systems seems well worth the effort of structuring these experiences. Open-ended groups deserve further conceptual clarification and research attention to support social work practice efforts.

NOTES

1. In our review of the social work, group therapy, and behavioral science literature, we found that most of the articles were primarily descriptive (see Bibliography). Our discussions with practitioners greatly facilitated our conceptualization of open-ended groups and we appreciate their willingness to share their experience with us.

2. H. J. Grosz and C. S. Wright, "The Tempo of Verbal Interaction in an Open Therapy Group Conducted in Rotation by Three Different Therapists," *International Journal of Group Psychotherapy*, 17 (October 1967), pp. 513-523; W. F. Hill and L. A. Gruner, "Study of Development in Open and Closed Groups," *Small Group Behavior*, 4 (August 1973), pp. 355-381; E. L. Hoch and G. Kaufer, "A Process Analysis of 'Transient' Therapy Groups," *International Journal of Group Psychotherapy*, 5 (October 1955), pp. 415-421; and, R. C. Ziller, "Toward a Theory of Open and Closed Groups," *Psychological Bulletin*, 64 (September 1965), pp. 164-182.

3. S. Bailis et al., "The Legacy of the Group: A Study of Group Therapy with a Transient Membership," *Social Work in Health Care*, 3 (Summer 1978), pp. 405-418; R. Paradise, "The Factor of Timing in the Addition of New Members to Established Groups," *Child Welfare*, 47 (November 1968), pp. 524-529, 553; and, B. Sadock et al., "Short-Term Group Psychotherapy in a Psychiatric Walk-In Clinic," *American Journal of Orthopsychiatry*, 38 (July 1968), pp. 724-732.

4. Our review of the social work, group therapy, and behavioral science literature on open-ended groups (see Bibliography) covers the period from 1970-1980 with inclusion of a few significant contributions prior to 1970. In addition to articles focused

on descriptions or beginning conceptualizations of open-ended groups, we reviewed articles on co-therapy and hospital groups which mentioned or described characteristics of open-ended groups. Further, we found a few articles on self-help that elaborated on the open-ended quality of these groups. The framework we have developed is directed toward professionals who lead open-ended groups but could be useful in consultation with self-help groups.

5. See, for example, H. Copeland, "The Beginning Group," *International Journal of Group Psychotherapy*, 30 (April 1980), pp. 201-212.

6. Although many authors refer to open-ended groups as an ongoing, available source of support, it is impossible to determine how frequently members return. Dube et al. indicate that in one of their six groups, all members were specifically given the option to return but only one came back for more than a "keep in touch visit." See B. D. Dube et al., "Uses of the Self-Run Group in a Child Guidance Setting," *International Journal of Group Psychotherapy*, 30 (October 1980), p. 474.

7. See I. M. Lesser and C. T. H. Friedman. "Beyond Medications: Group Therapy for the Chronic Psychiatric Patient," *International Journal of Group Psychotherapy*, 30 (April 1980), pp. 187-199; and, C. O. Levine and G. C. Dang. "The Group within the Group: The Dilemma of Cotherapy," *International Journal of Group Psychotherapy*, 29 (April 1979), pp. 175-184.

8. See A. Brooks, "Group Work on the Bowery," *Social Work with Groups*, 1 (Spring 1978), pp. 53-63; and, I. Weisman, "A Natural Group as a Vehicle for Change," *Social Work with Groups*, 1 (Winter 1978), pp. 355-363.

9. Scher found that it took the group about as long to adapt to a change in therapists as to membership change. See M. Scher, "Observations in an Aftercare Group," *International Journal of Group Psychotherapy*, 23 (July 1973), pp. 322-337.

10. J. Gotland, "A 'Hello' and 'Goodbye' Group," *International Journal of Group Psychotherapy*, 22 (April 1972), p. 258.

11. Our review of purposes reported in the literature on open-ended groups indicated that the frequency with which these purposes were mentioned, either singly or in combination, varied. Almost half of the articles reviewed cited coping with transition or crisis as a group purpose. Therapy, support, as well as screening and assessment were mentioned with almost equal frequency, and each was cited as a group purpose in about a quarter of the articles; educating clients, training and supervising staff, and outreach were rarely mentioned as purposes.

12. B. S. Comstock and M. McDermott, "Group Therapy for Patients Who Attempt Suicide," *International Journal of Group Psychotherapy*, 25 (January 1975), pp. 44-49.

13. L. C. Mone, "Short-Term Group Psychotherapy with Post-Cardiac Patients," *International Journal of Group Psychotherapy*, 20 (January 1970), pp. 99-108.

14. N. E. Kaltreider and L. D. Lenkoski, "Effective Use of Group Techniques in a Maternity Home," *Child Welfare*, 49 (March 1970), pp. 146-151.

15. Schwartz identifies the characteristics, modes of functioning, and problems of leadership in groups formed to deal with stressful life situations. His conceptualization of these groups is applicable to the many open-ended groups formed for this purpose. See M. O. Schwartz, "Situation/Transition Groups: A Conceptualization and Review," *American Journal of Orthopsychiatry*, 45 (October 1975), pp. 744-755.

16. The more specific delineations of transitions or crises under each category of purposes related to life stresses were obtained from our review of the literature. In

many cases, such as helping relatives deal with the illness of a family member, there was more than one report of an open-ended group serving this purpose.

17. Schwartz, pp. 746-748.

18. Collard, pp. 258-261.

19. For descriptions of open-ended groups with a psychotherapeutic orientation, see, for example, E. L. Edelstein and P. Noy, "Open Groups within a Changing Psychiatric Ward in Israel," *International Journal of Group Psychotherapy*, 22 (July 1972), pp. 379-383; J. Fleischer and C. Capellari, "Benefits of Co-Therapy in a Group with Schizophrenic Patients," *Group Analysis*, 12 (August 1979), pp. 117-126; H. J. Grosz and C. S. Wright, "The Tempo of Verbal Interaction in an Open Therapy Group Conducted in Rotation by Three Different Therapists," *International Journal of Group Psychotherapy*, 17 (October 1967), pp. 513-523; A. Manikoff, "Long-Term Psychotherapy with Puerto Rican Women: Ethnicity as a Clinical Support," *Group*, 3 (Fall 1979), pp. 172-180; J. Rosenburg and T. Cherbuliez, "Inpatient Group Therapy for Older Children and Pre-Adolescents," *International Journal of Group Psychotherapy*, 29 (July 1979), pp. 393-405; R. Shapiro, "Working Through the War with Vietnam Vets," *Group*, 2 (Fall 1978), pp. 156-183; and, D. S. Whitaker. "Some Conditions for Effective Work with Groups," *British Journal of Social Work*, 5 (Winter 1975), pp. 423-439.

20. Groups pursuing therapeutic purposes with a more present-oriented approach such as problem-solving are described in F. Canter, "A Self-Help Project with Hospitalized Alcoholics," *International Journal of Group Psychotherapy*, 19 (January 1969), pp. 16-27; J. K. Haaken and F. B. Davis, "Group Therapy with Latency-Age Psychotic Children," *Child Welfare*, 54 (December 1975), pp. 703-711; and, J. Williams et al., "A Model for Short-Term Group Therapy on a Children's Inpatient Unit," *Clinical Social Work Journal*, 6 (Spring 1978), pp. 21-32.

21. Whitaker, pp. 423-439.

22. See Dube et al., pp. 461-479; and, Levine and Dang, pp. 175-184.

23. For examples of screening groups, see E. F. Canton and E.1. Rawlings, "A Procedure for Orienting New Members to Group Psychotherapy," *Small Group Behavior*, 6 (August 1975), pp. 293-307; and, C. H. Hodgman and W. H. Stewart, "The Adolescent Screening Group," *International Journal of Group Psychotherapy*, 22 (April 1972), pp. 177-185.

24. See, for example, N. D. Bloom and J. G. Lynch, "Group Work in a Hospital Waiting Room," *Health and Social Work*, 4 (August 1979), pp. 48-63.

25. Copeland, pp. 201-212.

26. R. Roth, "A Transactional Analysis Group in Residential Treatment of Adolescents," *Child Welfare*, 56 (January 1977), pp. 776-786.

27. Golland, pp. 258-261; B. Stuckey et al., "Group Supervision of Student Companions to Psychotic Children," *International Journal of Group Psychotherapy*, 21 (July 1971), pp. 301-309; and, Williams et al., pp. 30-31.

28. Although average attendance is only discussed in some accounts of open-ended groups, consultation with practitioners supports the range indicated in the literature and confirms the need to be prepared for occasional meetings with only one or two members present. Average attendance is reported by Bailis et al., p. 407, who report 1-10 members; P. R. Balgopal and R. P. Hull, "Keeping Secrets: Group Resistance for Patients and Therapists," *Psychotherapy: Theory, Research and Practice*, 10 (Winter 1973), p. 334, who report an average of 6 members; Bloom and Lynch, p. 51, who report from 2-20 relatives attending their waiting-room group; A. B. Druck, "The Role of

Didactic Group Psychotherapy in Short-Term Psychiatric Settings," *Group*, 2 (Summer 1978), pp. 100 and 103, who reports 5-10 members in one group and 6-10 in a second group; Hoch and Kaufer, p. 415, who report from 10-20 members in attendance; Sadock et al.. p. 726, who report 2-8 members attending; Scher, p. 323. who reports 6-12 members attending over 90 percent of meetings; and, Williams et al., p. 23., who report 4 or 5 children typically at each session.

29. Bloom and Lynch, p. 56; Copeland, p. 209. Although not discussed in the literature, it may be helpful to invite reluctant members to observe a session before making a decision about membership, since exposure to the group experience may overcome negative attitudes and denial.

30. See L. H. Levy, "Self-Help Groups: Types and Psychological Processes," *Journal of Applied Behavioral Sciences*, 12 (July-August-September 1976), p. 315; and, Sadock et al., p. 730.

31. Scher reports that 230 patients used the aftercare group over a ten-year period. The average member remained for 20 sessions; two came for 80 sessions; and, some dropped out after only one session. In a number of cases, members did not attend continuously but returned after leaving the group. See Scher, pp. 325-329.

32. Grosz and Wright reported patients' average attendance was 5.5 sessions with a range of 1-23 sessions attended. See Grosz and Wright, p. 514.

33. Bloom and Lynch indicate members typically attended for a few days, but a few were present for up to two weeks. See Bloom and Lynch, p. 53.

34. Copeland reported that 75 percent attended all six sessions. See Copeland, pp. 202 and 212.

35. Ten of the twenty-eight members (35 percent) remained for all of the sessions. See Sadock et al., p. 726.

36. Ibid., p. 731.

37. Paradise draws on Garland, Jones, and Kolodny's stages of development and provides illustrations from children's groups. See Paradise, pp. 524-529 and 553.

38. Dube et al., pp. 470-474.

39. Scher, pp. 328 and 332.

40. Ziller, pp. 177-180.

41. Hill and Grimes, p. 381; and, Bailis et al., pp. 414-415.

42. J. R. Singler, "Group Work with Hospitalized Stroke Patients," *Social Casework*, 56 (June 1975), pp. 354.

43. T. J. Powell, "The Use of Self-Help Groups as Supportive Reference Communities," *American Journal of Orthopsychiatry*, 45 (October 1975), pp. 756-764.

44. Dube et al., p. 474.

45. Williams et al., pp. 26-28.

46. In a very early account of open-ended groups, Hoch and Kaufer identified four stages of development following the entry of a new member in an open-ended group but stressed that these might really represent the initial phases of more complete processes in stable, longer-term groups. See Hoch and Kaufer, p. 421.

47. Bailis et al., pp. 408-409; Copeland. pp. 204-209; and, Grosz and Wright, p. 517.

48. Hill and Gruner, pp. 375-380.

49. Scher, pp. 326-329.

50. Ziller, pp. 165-169.

51. Balgopal and Hull, pp. 334-336.

52. Singler, p. 354.

53. Sadock et al., p. 727.

54. Bailis et al., p. 414; Grosz and Wright, p. 519; and, Sadock et al., p. 728.
55. Bailis et al., pp. 414 and 418; and, Bloom and Lynch, p. 59.
56. Scher, pp. 336-337; and, Williams et al., pp. 23-24.
57. Bailis et al., pp. 413-414; and, Druck, p. 108.
58. For a description of each of Schwartz's phases of group development, see W. Schwartz, "On the Use of Groups in Social Work Practice," in W. Schwartz and S. R. Zalba (eds.), *The Practice of Group Work* (New York: Columbia University Press, 1971), pp. 13-18.
59. Sarri and Galinsky's framework for group development includes seven phases: Origin, Formative, Intermediate I, Revision, Intermediate II, Maturation, and Termination. In open-ended groups, the group may encounter a revision phase each time new members are added and/or old members leave. As the group repeats cycles through the revision and intermediate phases, it may gradually develop more and more characteristics of the mature group. Some open-ended groups may, however, never attain full maturity. For a description of these phases and the accompanying treatment sequence see, R. C. Sarri and M. J. Galinsky, "A Conceptual Framework for Group Development," In P. Glasser, R. Sarri and R. Vinter (eds.), *Individual Change Through Small Groups* (New York: The Free Press, 1974) pp. 71-88.

BIBLIOGRAPHY

Abramson, M. "Group Treatment of Families of Burn-Injured Patients." *Social Casework*, 56 (April 1975), pp. 235-241.

Abramson, R. M., Hoffman, L., and Johns, C. A. "Play Group Psychotherapy for Early Latency-Age Children on an Inpatient Psychiatric Unit." *International Journal of Group Psychotherapy*, 29 (July 1979), pp. 383-392.

Allgeyer, G. M. "The Crisis Group: Its Unique Usefulness to the Disadvantaged." *International Journal of Group Psychotherapy*, 20 (April 1970), pp. 235-240.

Asimos, C, T. "Dynamic Problem-Solving in a Group for Suicidal Persons." *International Journal of Group Psychotherapy*, 29 (January 1979), pp. 109-114.

Bailis, S., Lambert, S., and Bernstein, S. "The Legacy of the Group: A Study of Group Therapy with a Transient Membership." *Social Work in Health Care*, 3 (Summer 1978), pp. 405-418.

Balgopal, P. R., and Hull, R. F. "Keeping Secrets: Group Resistance for Patients and Therapists." *Psychotherapy: Theory, Research and Practice*, 10 (Winter 1973), pp. 334-336.

Barclay, L. "A Group Approach to Young, Unwed Mothers," *Social Casework*, 50 (July 1969), pp. 379-384.

Beck, L., Lattimer, J. K., and Brawn, E. "Group Psychotherapy on a Children's Urology Service." *Social Work in Health Care*, 4 (Spring 1979), pp. 275-285.

Bennett. L. "Group Service for COPD Out-Patients: Surmounting the Obstacles." *Social Work with Groups*, 2 (Spring 1979), pp. 145-160.

Bloom, N. D., and Lynch, J. G. "Group Work in a Hospital Waiting Room." *Health and Social Work*, 4 (August 1979), pp. 48-63.

Bolen, J. "Easing the Pain of Termination for Adolescents." *Social Casework*, 53 (November 1972), pp. 519-527.

Brooks, A. "Group Work on the Bowery." *Social Work with Groups*, I (Spring 1978), pp. 53-63.

Canter, F. "A Self-Help Project with Hospitalized Alcoholics." *International Journal of Group Psychotherapy*, 19 (January 1969), pp. 16-27.

Caterers, S. S. "Group Meetings for Families of Burned Children," *Health and Social Work*, 3 (August 1978), pp. 165-172.

Cheo, C. "Experiences with Group Psychotherapy in Taiwan," *International Journal of Group Psychotherapy*, 22 (April 1972), pp. 210-227.

Comstock, B. S., and McDermott, M. "Group Therapy for Patients Who Attempt Suicide." *International Journal of Group Psychotherapy*, 25 (January 1975), pp. 44-49.

Copeland, H. "The Beginning Group." *International Journal of Group Psychotherapy*, 30 (April 1980), pp. 201-212.

Crandall, R. "The Assimilation of Newcomers into Groups." *Small Group Behavior*, 9 (May 1978), pp. 331-336.

Cumiskey, P. A., and Mudd, H. P. "Postpartum Group Therapy with Unwed Mothers." *Child Welfare*, 51 (April 1972), pp. 241-246.

Daehlin, D., and Hynes, J. "A Mother's Discussion Group in a Women's Prison." *Child Welfare*, 53 (July 1974), pp. 464-470.

Davis. J. "Outpatient Group Therapy with Schizophrenic Patients." *Social Casework*, 52 (March 1971), pp. 172-178.

Driscoll, C., and Lubin. A. H. "Conferences with Parents of Children with Cystic Fibrosis." *Social Casework*, 53 (March 1972), pp. 140-146.

Druck, A. "The Role of Didactic Group Psychotherapy in Short-Term Psychiatric Settings." *Group*, 2 (Summer 1978), pp. 98-109.

Dube, B. D., Mitchell, C. A., and Bergman, L. A. "Uses of the Self-Run Group in a Child Guidance Setting." *International Journal of Group Psychotherapy*, 30 (October 1980), pp. 461-479.

Edelstein, E. L., and Noy, P. "Open Groups Within a Changing Psychiatric Ward in Israel." *International Journal of Group Psychotherapy*, 22 (July 1972), pp. 379-383.

Euster, S. "Rehabilitation after Mastectomy: The Group Process." *Social Work in Health Care*, 4 (Spring 1979), pp. 251-263.

Fielding, J., Guy, L., Harry, M., and Hook, R. H. "A Therapy Group Observed by Medical Students." *International Journal of Group Psychotherapy*, 21 (October 1971), pp. 467-488.

Fleischer, J., and Capellari, C. "Benefits of Co-Therapy in a Group with Schizophrenic Patients." *Group Analysis*, 12 (August 1979), pp. 117-126.

Foster, Z., and Mendel, S. "Mutual-Help Group for Patients: Taking Steps Toward Change." *Health and Social Work*, 4 (August 1979), pp. 82-98.

Gauren, E. F., and Raulings, E. I. "A Procedure for Orienting New Members to Group Psychotherapy." *Small Group Behavior*, 6 (August 1975), pp. 293-307.

Golland, J. "A 'Hello' and 'Goodbye' Group." *International Journal of Group Psychotherapy*, 22 (April 1972), pp. 258-261.

Grosz, H. J., and Wright, C. S. "The Tempo of Verbal Interaction in an Open Therapy Group Conducted in Rotation by Three Different Therapists." *International Journal of Group Psychotherapy*, 17 (October 1967), pp. 513-523.

Haaken, J. K., and Davis, F, B. "Group Therapy with Latency-Age Psychotic Children." *Child Welfare*, 54 (December 1975), pp. 703-711.

Harris, P. B. "Being Old: A Confrontation Group with Nursing Home Residents." *Health and Social Work*, 4 (February 1979), pp. 152-166.

Hartford, M. E. "Groups in Human Services: Some Facts and Fancies." *Social Work with Groups*, 1 (Spring 1978), pp. 7-13.

Hendricks, W. J. "Use of Multifamily Counseling Groups in Treatment of Male Narcotic Addicts." *International Journal of Group Psychotherapy*, 21 (January 1971), pp. 84-90.

Henkle, C. "Social Group Work as a Treatment Modality for Hospitalized People with Rheumatoid Arthritis." *Rehabilitative Literature*, 36 (November 1975), pp. 334-341.

Herstein, N., and Simon, N. "A Group Model Lot Residential Treatment." *Child Welfare*, 56 (November 1977), pp. 601-611.

Hill, W. F., and Gruner, L. A. "Study of Development in Open and Closed Groups." *Small Group Behavior*, 4 (August 1973), pp. 355-381.

Hoch, E. L., and Kaufer, G. "A Process Analysis of 'Transient' Therapy Groups," *International Journal of Group Psychotherapy*, 5 (October 1955), pp. 415-421.

Hodgman, C. H., and Stewart, W. H. "The Adolescent Screening Group." *International Group Psychotherapy*, 22 (April 1972), pp. 177-185.

Holmes, S. "Parents Anonymous: A Treatment Method for Child Abuse," *Social Work*, 23 (May 1978), pp. 245-247.

Irwin, S., and Lloyd-Stilt, D. "The Use of Groups to Mobilize Strengths During Hospitalization of Children." *Child Welfare*, 53 (May 1974), pp. 305-312.

Kaltreider, N. B., and Lenkoski, L. D. "Effective Use of Group Techniques in a Maternity Home." *Child Welfare*, 49 (March 1970), pp. 146-151.

Kate, A. H. "Self-Help Groups and the Professional Community." *The Social Welfare Forum*. New York: Columbia University Press, 1976, pp. 142-153.

Katz, A. "Self-Help Organizations and Volunteer Participation in Social Welfare." *Social Work*, 15 (January 1970), pp. 51-60.

La Vorgna, D. "Group Treatment for Wives of Patients with Alzheimer's Disease." *Social Work in Health Care*, 5 (Winter 1979), pp. 219-221.

Lesser, I. M., and Friedman, C. T. H. "Beyond Medications: Group Therapy for the Chronic Psychiatric Patient," *International Journal of Group Psychotherapy*, 30 (April 1980), pp. 187-199.

Levine, B., and Schild, J. "Group Treatment of Depression." *Social Work*, 14 (October 1969), pp. 46-52.

Levine. C. O., and Deng, G. C. "The Group Within the Group: The Dilemma of Cotherapy." *International Journal of Group Psychotherapy*, 29 (April 1979), pp. 175-184.

Levinson, V. L. "The Decision Groups: Beginning Treatment in an Alcoholism Clinic." *Health and Social Work*, 4 (Summer 1979), pp. 199-221.

Levy, L. H. "Self Help Groups: Types and Psychological Processes." *Journal of Applied Behavioral Sciences*, 12 (July-August-September 1976), pp. 310-322.

Lubell, A. "Group Work with Patients on Peritoneal Dialysis." *Health and Social Work*, 1 (August 1976), pp. 158-176.

Macon, L. B. "Help for Bereaved Parents." *Social Casework*, 60 (November 1979), pp. 558-561.

Meier, G. "A Health-Oriented Program for Emotionally Disturbed Women." *Social Casework*, 56 (July 1975), pp. 411-417.

Menikoff, A. "Long-Term Psychotherapy with Puerto Rican Women: Ethnicity as a Clinical Support." *Group,* 3 (Fall 1979), pp. 172-180.

Mone, L. C. "Short-Term Group Psychotherapy with Post-Cardiac Patients." *International Journal of Group Psychotherapy*, 20 (January 1970), pp. 99-108.

Murphy, A., Siegfried, M. P., and Schneider, J. "Group Work with Parents of Children with Down's Syndrome." *Social Casework*, 54 (February 1973), pp. 114-119.

O'Connor, A. "A Creative Living Center for Mentally Ill." *Social Casework*, 51 (November 1970), pp. 544-550.

Oradei, D. M., and Waite, N. S. "Group Psychotherapy with Stroke Patients During the Immediate Recovery Phase." *American Journal of Orthopsychiatry*, 44 (April 1974), pp. 386-395.

Page, R. C. "Developmental Stages of Unstructured Counseling Groups with Prisoners." *Small Group Behavior*, 10 (May 1979), pp. 271-278.

Paradise, R. "The Factor of Timing in the Addition of New Members to Established Groups." *Child Welfare*, 47 (November 1968), pp. 524-529, 553.

Parry, J. K., and Kahn, N. "Group Work with Emphysema Patients." *Social Work in Health Care*, 2 (Fall 1976), pp. 55-64.

Powell, T. J. "Interpreting Parents Anonymous as a Source of Help for Those with Child Abuse Problems." *Child Welfare*, 58 (February 1979), pp. 105-114.

Powell, T. J. "The Use of Self-Help Groups as Supportive Reference Communities." *American Journal of Orthopsychiatry*, 45 (October 1975), pp. 756-764.

Rice, C. "Observations on the Unexpected and Simultaneous Termination of Leader and Group." *Group*, 1 (Summer 1977), pp. 110-117.

Rodewald, D. "Social Work with a Blind Group." *Health and Social Work*, 2 (November 1977), pp. 157-163.

Rosenburg, J., and Cherbuliez, T. "Inpatient Group Therapy for Older Children and Pre-Adolescents." *International Journal of Group Psychotherapy*, 29 (July 1979), pp. 393-405.

Roth, R. "A Transactional Analysis Group in Residential Treatment of Adolescents." *Child Welfare*, 56 (January 1977), pp. 776-786.

Rubin, S. "Parent's Group in a Psychiatric Hospital for Children." *Social Work*, 23 (September 1978), pp. 416-417.

Sadock, B., Newman, L., and Normand, W. C. "Short-Term Group Psychotherapy in a Psychiatric Walk-In Clinic." *American Journal of Orthopsychiatry*, 38 (July 1968), pp. 724-732.

Samit, C., Nash. K., and Meyers, J. "The Parents Group: A Therapeutic Tool." *Social Casework*, 61 (April 1980), pp. 215-222.

Sands, P. M., and Hanson, P. G. "Psychotherapeutic Groups for Alcoholics and Relatives in an Outpatient Setting." *International Journal of Group Psychotherapy*, 21 (January 1971), pp. 23-33.

Sarri, R., and Galinsky, M. J. "A Conceptual Framework for Group Development," in P. Glasser, R. Sarri, and R. Vinter (eds.), *Individual Change Through Small Groups*. New York: The Free Press, 1974, pp. 71-88.

Schardt, E., and Truckle, B. "Notes on a Counseling Group for Adolescents." *Group Analysis*, 8 (December 1975), pp. 166-169.

Scher, M. "Observations in an Aftercare Group." *International Journal of Group Psychotherapy*, 23 (July 1973), pp. 322-337.

Schual, F., Sater, H., and Paley, M. G. "'Thematic' Group Therapy in the Treatment of Hospitalized Alcoholic Patients." *International Journal of Group Psychotherapy*, 21 (April 1971), pp. 226-233.

Schwartz, M. D. "Situation/Transition Groups: A Conceptualization and Review." *American Journal of Orthopsychiatry*, 45 (October 1975), pp. 744-755.

Schwartz, W. "On the Use of Groups in Social Work Practice," in W. Schwartz and S. R. Zalba (eds.), *The Practice of Group Work*. New York: Columbia University Press, 1971, pp. 3-24.

Shapiro, R. "Working Through the War with Vietnam Vets." *Group*, 2 (Fall 1978), pp. 156-183.

Sharpe, M. "Group Themes in a District General Hospital Psychiatric Unit-Schrodells, Watford, England." *Group Analysis*, 10 (December 1977), pp. 266-273.

Shore, J. "The Use of the Self-Identity Workshop with Recovering Alcoholics." *Social Work with Groups*, 1 (Fall 1978), pp. 299-307.

Singler, J. R. "Group Work with Hospitalized Stroke Patients." *Social Casework*, 56 (June 1975), pp. 348-354.

Smith, M. M. "Notes on a Therapeutic Non-Group." *Group Analysis*, 3 (August 1970), pp. 80-82.

Smith, O. S., and Gundlach, R. H. "Group Therapy for Blacks in a Therapeutic Communtty." *American Journal of Orthopsychiatry*, 44 (January 1974), pp. 26-36.

Spiegel, D., and Yalom, I. D. "A Support Group for Dying Patients." *International Journal of Group Psychotherapy*, 28 (April 1978), pp. 233-245.

Stuckey. B., Garrett, M. W., and Sugar, M. "Group Supervision of Student Companions to Psychotic Children." *International Journal of Group Psychotherapy*, 21 (July 1971), pp. 301-309.

Vatlano, A. "Power to the People: Self-Help Groups." *Social Work*, 17 (July 1972), pp. 7-15.

Weisman, I. "A Natural Group as a Vehicle for Change." *Social Work with Groups*, 1 (Winter 1978), pp. 355-363.

Wellisch D. K., Mosher, M. G., and Van Scoy, C. "Management of Family Emotion Stress: Family Group Therapy in a Private Oncology Practice." *International Journal of Group Psychotherapy*, 28 (April 1978), pp. 225-231.

Whitaker. D. S. "Some Conditions for Effective Work with Groups." *British Journal of Social Work*, 5 (Winter 1975), pp. 423-439.

Williams, J., Lewis, C., Copeland, F., Tucker, L., and Feagan, L. "A Model for Short-Term Group Therapy on a Children's Inpatient Unit." *Clinical Social Work Journal*, 6 (Spring 1978), pp. 21-32.

Ziller, R. C. "Toward a Theory of Open and Closed Groups." *Psychological Bulletin*, 64 (September 1965), pp. 164-182.

The Group Work Tradition
and Social Work Practice

William Schwartz

The social work profession is one of the primary institutions designed to help people negotiate the complicated systems in which they live. Its efforts have followed three major impulses. The most prominent of these has been to deal with people individually, "case by case," seeking to remedy the psychological and social conditions that have brought their problems about. Theories of responsibility vary with the times–individual and social, moral, economic, and psychological–but in most instances those who seek help are seen as somehow personally inadequate, and the effort is made to render them more self-sufficient, psychologically stronger, less dependent on help from the outside. The worker-client relationship is intimate, confidential, and takes place on the professional's own ground. The client is carefully examined, and the condition "diagnosed"–in the adopted medical language–as a prelude to "treatment." The rationale for this thorough personal inquiry is today largely scientific, following the medical approach to illness. But the tra-

---

This paper was presented at the 25th Anniversary Symposia, Graduate School of Social Work, Rutgers, the State University of New Jersey, and is republished with permission from *Social Work Futures: Essays Commemorating Twenty-Five Years of the Graduate School of Social Work*, edited by Miriam Dinerman, published by the Graduate School of Social Work, Rutgers, The State University of New Jersey in cooperation with the Council on Social Work Education, 1983, New Brunswick, NJ.

This article was originally published in *Social Work with Groups*, Vol. 8 (4), 1985/86.

[Haworth co-indexing entry note]: "The Group Work Tradition and Social Work Practice." Schwartz. William. Co-published simultaneously in *Social Work with Groups* (The Haworth Press, Inc.) Vol. 28, No. 3/4, 2005, pp. 69-89; and: *A Quarter Century of Classics (1978-2004): Capturing the Theory, Practice, and Spirit of Social Work with Groups* (ed: Andrew Malekoff, and Roselle Kurland) The Haworth Press, Inc., 2005, pp. 69-89. Single or multiple copies of this article are available for a fee from The Haworth Document Delivery Service [1-800-HAWORTH, 9:00 a.m. - 5:00 p.m. (EST). E-mail address: docdelivery@haworthpress.com].

Available online at http://www.haworthpress.com/web/SWG
doi:10.1300/J009v28n03_06

dition goes back a long way. Thomas Chalmers, an early precursor of the Charity Organization movement, said of those who came to seek economic assistance: "He who seeks another's bounty shall also submit to another's scrutiny."[1] This one-on-one approach to human problems is the discipline we have called social casework, and it has been the dominant feature of the social work profession since its inception.

A second direction has been to help needy people in their own milieux, surrounded by their peers and working in an atmosphere of mutual aid. Here the effort is to find, in the people's own conditions of life, the energy and the resources with which they can help each other act together on common problems. People are brought together for many reasons: to organize themselves for action on special interests and common concerns; to help each other face difficult personal problems; to learn new skills with which to enrich the quality of their lives. The setting is the small, face-to-face group, placed in some shared community context; experiences are communicated among the members, rather than held confidential between member and worker; and the worker is surrounded by a host of surrogate helpers, each claiming a share of the supportive function. The lines of communication are intricate, and the worker's authority is diffused in the network of relationships that goes to make up the pattern of mutual aid. This is the direction we came to know as social group work, and it has grown over the years to occupy an increasingly significant place in the work of the profession.

The third approach has been to deal with the social problems themselves, rather than the people who suffer under their effects. The lines between direct service and social planning have not always been distinct, nor has it been necessary that they be so. In fact, both the early settlements and the Charity Organization movement were prime examples of the integration of direct practice and what we now call community organization and social reform. But the deepening troubles of industrial capitalism, and the accompanying complexities administering social welfare, created this specialized field, with its own knowledge and skills, that addressed itself to the tasks of social and legislative action, the development and distribution of resources, intergroup cooperation, and–maintaining its ties to direct service–the organization of grass-roots action on community problems.

The history of social work is the story of how these different ways of helping people in need came together to find a single professional identity. In 1873, the National Conference of Charities and Correction first offered the humanitarians a chance to share their common aspirations and working problems.[2] In the 1920s, the Milford Conference found some theoretical unity for social casework, at a time when that was considered tantamount to integrating the entire profession.[3] And in the 1950s, the National Association of Social Workers was born of a long organizational process that merged seven independent social work organizations into a single association that represented social workers of America who had formal educational preparation.[4,5]

The search for a common identity for social work did not end when this union was effected. Today, a generation later, it still remains to find the common technology that could render its practitioners recognizable as part of a single professional entity. It has been relatively easy to describe the common objectives, the shared values, even the relevant areas of knowledge; but it has been much more difficult to define the basic skills that bind them together and constitute a special claim to competence in serving the community. Parsons, in his study of the legal profession, defined the professional as a "technical expert . . . by virtue of his mastery of the tradition and skills of its use."[6] How would such a principle be applied to social work? What is its common tradition, and to what special skills does it lay its claim? What abilities do the family worker, the camp director, the organizer, the club leader, the clinician-therapist have in common? Are they in any measure interchangeable, considering that they all hold the same graduate degree?

It is, of course, the old search for the generic, in a jungle of specifics. The merger of professional associations, however desirable it may have been, left yet to be done the task of merging the separate experiences and histories of social work into a commonly understood way of working with people. Although structurally unified, the profession is still more like a coalition of the old "methods" than it is an integrated discipline combining the richest and most effective elements of each.

It is true that such development does not happen overnight; the Milford Conference, for example, took close to a decade to sort out the generic and the specific in social casework. In our own generation, we have had some thoughtful work on the subject,[7,8] and there will be more. But I believe that such an effort would be considerably advanced if each of the so-called "methods" were to explore its own traditions of practice to find those unique elements that might help to put its own special stamp on a unified conception of the function and practice of social work. My effort here is to examine something of the group work heritage, looking back on some of its early history, its theoretical underpinnings, its conception of the client, the worker-member relationship, and its conduct of the helping process. In a short paper, one can only touch on the main themes; but one would hope to give some of the flavor of such an enterprise, and stimulate others to work along similar lines.[9]

The Early Years

There is a common misconception that group work is considerably younger than its casework sibling. In fact, the ancestors of both movements began their work at about the same time in history, with the group work agencies following the casework establishments by only a few years. Canon Barnett, the founder of the first settlement–Toynbee Hall in London–was a close associate of Octavia Hill, who played a similar role in the beginnings of the London Charity Organization Society; Barnett was in fact influential in both movements.[10] In this country, Jane Addams and Mary Richmond were colleagues and very much aware that they were part of a common enterprise. Both in England and in the United States, the settlements and the Societies were not far apart: the London COS in 1868, Toynbee Hall in 1884, the Buffalo COS in 1877, Jane Addams's Hull-House in 1889. As to the seminal works in both fields, Mary Richmond's *Social Diagnosis* was issued in 1917,[11] while Grace Coyle's *Social Process in Organized Groups* came in 1930.[12] In general, the early workers were all part of the same group of social reformers that came out of the Progressive Era. Their motives were much the same, and they knew and worked with each other long before the casework-group work distinctions were drawn. Canon Barnett's favored motto–embroidered and hung in his drawing room in Whitechapel–was "One By One."[13]

The historical difference between the two movements was that casework, or individual work, became almost immediately synonymous with social work as its practitioners sprang into action, defined themselves as a body, formed a national conference, began to systematize their thinking,[14] and produced a steady stream of writing about their experiences in the field. The group workers, on the other hand, were much more diverse in their outlook, identifying themselves with many fields of endeavor, among them education, recreation, camping, and mental hygiene–each with a tradition of its own going back to 1861[15]–as well as social work. The American Association for the Study of Group Work, founded in 1936, numbered among its members people from all these professions, as well as those with purely academic and scientific interest in the small group, without any particular reference to its professional uses.

This wide range of interests and allegiances was reflected in a study of the leisure-time agencies in the 1920s, which concluded that "the objectives of these various agencies would at first thought seem so divergent as to make it impossible to treat the duties and responsibilities of their workers in the same analysis."[16]

Group work's ambivalence about where it belonged continued even after its place was established, both in social work education and as part of the National Conference of Social Work, in the mid-30s. In 1940, the noted educator William Heard Kilpatrick asserted that "this group work is . . . not to be thought of as a separate field of work, but rather as a method to be used in all kinds of educational effort."[17] And as late as 1946, we find Grace Coyle herself still concerned about the "alignment" of group workers: "One baffling problem has plagued the development of professional consciousness among group workers over this decade. It is usually phrased in terms of alignment, and a dilemma is presented. We must, it seems, be either educators or social workers."[18]

Ultimately, the choice was made, and group work practitioners found their place within the social work profession. It was, after all, group work's natural habitat, having had its origins in the humanitarian movement and its major development within the agencies of social welfare.

> Social work, with its early emphasis on the individual in his environment, was a congenial host for those whose work lay at the very point of interaction between the two. Social work's concern with the total individual, the importance of community life, and the role of government in human affairs offered a comfortable resting place for group work's unique blend of scientific, humanitarian, and missionary zeal. . . .[19]

It was at that point that the question changed from whether group workers would identify themselves as social workers to what they would bring with them into a unified field of practice. Undoubtedly, there was much in their world view that was the same as that of the other approaches within the profession. But there must also be, from the settings and circumstances of their encounters with human beings in need, a great deal that was different, through which group work could make a valuable contribution to a generic conception of the work of the profession. To find these, one would have to look closely at several key areas in their collective early experience.

Group Work Purposes

If the caseworkers were the "priests" of social welfare, and the social planners were its "prophets," the group workers were a kind of cross between the two.[20] On the one hand, they were deeply involved in direct service to the poor, ministering to their needs in day-to-day contact; on the other, because they worked where the people lived, they were first-hand witnesses to the cramped quality of the people's lives and the limitations of a political and economic system in which huge sections of the population were neglected, uninvolved, and relegated to the fringes of power. Catherine Cooke Gilman suggested that the motto of the settlements might be: "Keep your fingers on the near things and eyes on the far things."[21]

These were the twin emphases that pervaded the work of the first agencies–the "near things" of individual need and the "far things" of social reform. On the one hand, the early settlement papers were replete with references to "self": self-development, self-sufficiency, self-respect, and the like.[22] At the same time, there was a strong preoccupation with the need for education for political power. "If power is to be dispersed, then everybody is to be trained to exercise it. . . . Democracy becomes a farce, not because it has lost its ideal force but because its devotees are, democratically speaking, illiterate; they do not know how to operate in and through groups."[23]

In order to provide a new version of society, a community in which people could regain some control over their immediate environment, the early workers turned to the small group as a context for action. This connection between individual and social strength may seem naive to us today, but it appeared to the settlement pioneers to be compelling; they had an enormous faith in human association, and the small group was to be an instrument of personal growth as well as what they called a "building block of democracy." Jane Addams spoke of exchanging "the music of isolated voices [for] the volume and strength of the chorus."[24] And Canon Barnett said: ". . . if it be a great matter to be an individual, it is a greater matter to be part of a whole . . ."[25]

Underlying all of these purposes, there lay the urge to restore to the people those aspects of life that had been denied to them by the ravages of industrialization. The crowded city streets, the dearth of recreational opportunities, the absence of trees and country spaces, the lack of time for play–all of these produced a great yearning for space, country, and leisure. It was the need that spawned Barnett's Children's Country Holiday Fund in England, and vitalized the camping and playground movements in this country. The group work pioneers waxed particularly eloquent on the subject of play. "A people's play," said Mrs. Henrietta Barnett, "is a fair test of a people's character. Their recreation more than their business or their conquests settle the nations' place in history."[26] And consider this paean to its virtues:

> Play has physical, psychological, social, ethical, and spiritual significance.... Play is joy-producing and hence develops mental optimism. Play naturally and unconsciously places the individual in right relations with his social group. Play is the testing-laboratory of the individual and the social virtues. Play rounds out our fragmentary lives and makes us spiritually whole.[27]

This concern with enhancing the quality of life was at the heart of the preoccupation with cultural activities–music, art, literature, drama, trips, discussion–as well as occasions, entertainments, and general atmosphere of intimate and informal exchange. Barnett claimed that his ultimate resource was his wife's tea-table.[28] The themes of informality, social intercourse, shared experience, and, above all, friendship, were at the very roots of the settlement movement. Friendship was the bond that would unite them all–the residents and the neighbors, workers and members. Indeed friendship was to be a political instrument. The young, well-favored, well-to-do students who came to the first university settlements–of which Toynbee Hall was one–were being trained to rule more wisely by making real friendships with the poor and learning at first hand their way of life. The class struggle was in their eyes a product of misunderstanding between the rich and the poor, and it could be mitigated by working out these failures of communication on the people's home ground. "The classes are out of joint," wrote Barnett "and do not work together to one end. The call is still for a way of peace, and for a means of promoting good fellowship between man and man."[29]

And so group work came to the people with an active agenda and a sackful of hopes and prayers for individual salvation and social change. Although Barnett himself went to some pains to point out that settlements are not missions, and should not be used for "doing good," or for preaching a message,[30] the total effect over the years has been to invest the worker-client engagement with urgent conviction and well-marked educational purposes. Later, when "cause" began to edge its way toward "function," there would be considerable difficulty in distinguishing means from ends. But there was rarely any danger that the group workers would go passive, or neutral, about what the world should be like. They would carry their strong sense of the individual-social connections with them into the social work arena. It was a heavy load, and they often carried it clumsily; but always the worker was an active and intimate participant in the client's experience.

It was a new kind of relationship, this collaboration between a worker and the members of a group, and it raised questions that went beyond the Freudian explanations that were being studied so intently by the rest of the profession. Unbound as they were to any one field of exploration, they had a whole world to turn to; and they did—to the educators, the sociologists, the psychologists, and the host of disciplines that were exploding with new insights at the turn of the 20th century.

Theoretical Foundations

The intellectual renaissance that took place in America as part of the Progressive Era was in many ways responsive to the needs and curiosities of the group work movement. New knowledge came from many directions—religious, philosophical, social, psychological, political—and the group workers, not yet tied to any hard-and-fast identifications, were free to look where they chose for enlightenment and inspiration. The Freudian answers found some ready group work adherents, as they did in casework, but the fit was uncomfortable, the explanations skirting many of the situational questions raised by the group experience. It was not that the group workers had no interest in personality development; obviously they must have. But their point of vantage led them to observe human behavior in its social, relational context. Their curiosities were essentially what we would now call *systemic*, having to do with interrelational networks; and their questions were oriented to issues of action and interaction, the nature of shared experience, and the processes of communication—verbal and nonverbal—within the small group.

Their field of inquiry was broad, and it would take a much longer work than this to trace the precise connections between the growing body of early 20th century knowledge and the development of group work thinking. But certain influences are fairly clear, and important to our present purpose. The great progenitor of small-group analysis was, of course, Charles Horton Cooley, whose researches into the nature of the primary group provided a profound rationale for the social uses of human togetherness. It was Cooley who took his stand against the opposition of self and society, uniting these into a single, unified concept. He said: "By primary groups I mean those characterized by intimate face-to-face association and cooperation. They are primary in several senses, but chiefly in that they are fundamental in forming the social nature and ideals of the individual."[31] It was a radical idea, and it explained much of the group workers' experience with people. ". . . human nature is not something existing separately in the individual, but a *group-nature* . . ."[32] And he echoed another part of their experience as he described the feeling of "we": "one lives in the feeling of the whole and finds the chief aims of his will in that feeling."[33]

The concept of the social nature of human personality was a landmark in our intellectual history, and it was highly congenial to those who worked in the context of community. The group workers turned to others with the same idea–Baldwin,[34] Kropotkin,[35] and Dewey[36] in the early years, and later Mead,[37] Sherif,[38] Lewin,[39] and the host of others that followed. The implications of this insight moved directly to the heart of one of the great issues of group work practice, namely the persistent tendency to dichotomize the needs of individuals and those of the collective. Baldwin put it this way:

> It is, to my mind, the most remarkable outcome of modern social theory–the recognition of the fact that the individual's normal growth lands him in essential solidarity with his fellows, while on the other hand the exercise of his social duties and privileges advances his highest and purest individuality.[40]

Like all great insights, this one raised new questions to replace those it answered. How, for example, did one understand the processes of interaction between people who were not fixed entities but social creations, the ever-changing products of those same interactions? For this they turned to Mary Follett, an ex-settlement worker in working-class Boston, who wrote books analyzing the group experience, the uses of authority, the nature of freedom, and similar, eagerly debated, issues affecting group work practice. Her concept of "circular behavior" emphasized the *reverberating* character of human exchanges, in which each actor responds to a situation he helped create a moment ago. She pointed out that "response is always to a relation. I respond, not only to you, but to the relation between you and me."[41] This idea took on considerable meaning as workers tried to describe a helping process in which they did not attempt to change the fixed and immutable "personality" of their members, but viewed both client and worker as in a continuing process of shifting and changing under the moment-by-moment impact of each upon the other. In the spontaneous, ever-active ambience of the group experience, this latter version, however difficult to describe, was felt to be closer to experience than the subject-object, "change-agent," what Buber was later to call the "I-It" rather than the "I-Thou"[42] version of the helping process.

It was a day-by-day discovery of the group workers that communication was only partly a formal, verbal affair, and that much of the human exchange could be read in the language of action–in games, body language, and expressive play. In this area, their teacher was Neva Leona Boyd. Using her long experience as a pioneer of the recreation movement, and taking her cues from the literature of spontaneity and progressive education, she asserted that "the only morality there is is bound up with action."[43] She urged the group workers to free themselves "from the limitations imposed by an overemphasis on verbalized aspects of expression. "[44] And she said: "Only in the spontaneous, uncalculated response of human beings to each other can sensitivity to undefined subtleties function."[45]

There was a great deal more, and as the field moved into the '30s and '40s, it was Grace Coyle and her colleagues who pulled it all together and made it into a syllabus. The time for building their own theoretical base was getting short; there would be less than ten years between the formation of the American Association of Group Workers in 1946 and its merger into the National Association of Social Workers in 1955, and there were many important questions left to be resolved.

The Group Work Client

There are those who claim that all of social work is a kind of "battlefield medicine," in which the object is to patch up the victims as best one can and put them back in the field as soon as possible. If this is so, then the triage was arranged so that the group workers took those who were the less incapacitated and somewhat more capable of conducting their affairs as part of a small community. This is not to say, as it is so often, that their people were "normal"–there are so few of those around–but simply that they had enough energy to engage themselves with others in common tasks. The emphasis was on working with strengths, rather than curing illness. At the 1935 National Conference of Social Work, LeRoy Bowman said: "Group work . . . is not a service to those who ask for help–it is the social mechanism perfectly competent people utilize to achieve their own ends."[46] And just as Virginia Robinson had written that "one does not go to a [casework] agency joyfully,"[47] Grace Coyle stresses the "true enjoyment [that] comes when the self is . . . actively and vitally engaged, its powers expanding in fulfillment."[48]

Thus it was that the very concept of "client" was somewhat strange, even distasteful, for many group workers, preferring as they did the designation of "member." Bowman was careful to make a point of this at the same conference in 1935, asserting that group workers "must help to relate the members of their groups (I did not say 'clients') to the national or mass concerns of the day."[49] The argument about terms was, of course, part of the aforementioned ambivalence about social work itself; but it had a deeper significance in that the "member" orientation helped bring millions of new middle-class consumers into group work's field of action, as the group work skills were sought out by the youth movements, community centers, "Y"s, and Jewish Centers that were coming into being all over the country.

The distinction between "client" and "member" was not always easy to maintain; group workers were constantly dealing with group members who were struggling under a heavy load of personal problems as they tried to meet the demand for responsible group participation. Thus workers faced what came increasingly to feel like a choice between their concern for individuals in trouble and their aspirations for the group as a whole. Here again was the self-society dilemma in its practice manifestation: whether to get on with the collective tasks or to stop for those who needed help in catching up with the others. The "choice," though it was much discussed, always turned out to be an illusion, in the small group as in the larger community: when one "chose" the individual and abandoned the others, the group foundered and all suffered; and when the worker addressed himself exclusively to the collective, ignoring those who needed special help, there was a mounting residue of anger and guilt, felt by both members and worker.

Out of this dilemma there emerged what has been called the "two clients" conception, in which the worker's function is to help both the individual and the group, the one to meet his needs within the system, the other to pursue its collective tasks. The value of this idea was that it called for considerable skill and forced the worker to try to unify his responsibility for both the individual and the group, instead of hovering indecisively between the two, always worrying about whether he should be sacrificing one for the other.

But the trouble with the "two clients" idea was that it was still dualistic in nature. While "both" was superior to "either-or," it was really only a different version of it, and it tended to produce a kind of pseudo-solution that obscured a deeper insight into the problem. What was needed was a closer look at the working relationship between a person and his group, to find the common need, the common ground, the common impetus that carried them toward each other.[50] In this view, the worker's function was to act as a bridge across which the individual could reach out to negotiate the system of demands and opportunities offered by his group, while at the same time helping the collective reach out to incorporate each of its members in the group life.[51] The worker would thus define his "client"–or his major responsibility–as neither the individual nor the group, but the *processes* that passed between them. The group workers had learned about process from Dewey, Follett, Lindeman, and others; it was a natural outgrowth of their interest in social action and social experience. It was no accident that Coyle's first landmark publication was called *Social Process in Organized Groups*, while Mary Richmond's was entitled *Social Diagnosis*.

The group workers could not always muster the skills necessary to help carry people and their significant groups toward each other; the burden of process is not easy to carry in a product-oriented society. Nevertheless, operating where these problems were always right before their eyes, they could not but form the habit of viewing people in their social context. When they looked at an individual–be he "client" or "member"–they could not fail to see him as surrounded by his culture, his family, and his friends.

The Worker-Client Relationship

The earliest conception of the helping relationship in group work was of one that took place within a community of equals. As I have indicated, the theme of friendship was paramount in the minds of the founders: "Charity is friendship," said Canon Barnett, "and . . . institutions which don't give friends are not charity."[52] The Charity Organization Society also used the slogan "not alms but a friend,"[53] but the settlements used the term literally, and carried it into action with its daily opportunities for physical contact, joint action, group entertainments, and the like.

The theme of camaraderie–of comradeship as an instrument of helping–had a lasting effect on the development of the group work tradition. It became a subject of humor in the sophisticated fellowship into which it subsequently entered, but when the idea of friendship was later transformed into that of leadership, the group workers found themselves formulating an important problem in the uses of professional authority. How did one maintain an active, intimate, spontaneous relationship with a person in need, while yet retaining the distance and discipline necessary to carry out a professional function? How did a worker act freely without acting out?

Freud's discovery of the "transference" in the doctor-patient relationship[54] was a revelation to workers in the helping disciplines, and it was eagerly taken up by the newly emerging social work profession. He had written that "eventually all the conflicts must be fought out on the field of transference," and, in advising physicians on the use of the psychoanalytic method, he had laid great stress on the absolute "impenetrability" of the doctor in the face of this phenomenon:

> The loosening of the transference, too–one of the main tasks of the cure–is made more difficult by too intimate an attitude on the part of the doctor, so that a doubtful gain in the beginning is more than cancelled in the end. Therefore I do not hesitate to condemn this kind of technique as incorrect. The physician should be impenetrable to the patient, and, like a mirror, reflect nothing but what is shown to him.[56]

Obviously, such a doctrine, however useful in helping workers understand more deeply the meaning of professional authority, was difficult to apply directly in the hustle-bustle of the group experience. And, as we might expect, there was some horror at the prospect. Again it was Bowman who stated the problem:

> Any good group worker knows, as does any good progressive teacher, that such a relationship is the opposite of that desired by the group leader. It is not transference to the leader at all, but cross transference between the members, that should form the dynamic influence in group activities.[57]

In this area as in others, the group workers found the new, system-oriented ideas more congenial to their experience. While always troubled by their tendency towards counter-transference, and their vulnerability to its effects, it was difficult to remain "impenetrable" in a game of steal-the-bacon, or a trip to a strange place, or a discussion of serious group problems. But they could echo to Follett's description of the helping relationship as circular and reciprocal–"a reaction to a relating." And they could respond to her brilliant insight, realized as early as the '20s, that leadership was not essentially a factor of personality–what she called "ascendency traits"–but a functional, situational manifestation. "Don't exploit your personality," she said to them. "*Learn your job*."[58]

Later in their development, the group workers would be heavily in-fluenced by Grace Coyle's distillation of the educational process and her conception of the *mentoring* and *modelling* aspects of the profes-sional relationship.

> In this interacting mesh of life, whatever the content of program, teaching and learning are a mutual process. If the leader is himself achieving his own guiding values, his own delight in excellence, his own deep sense of the validity and meaning of life, his own ability to function as part of the social whole, that achieving by a kind of delicate osmosis is likely to be his most significant contri-bution to his group.[59]

Thus the traditional worker-member relationship in group work was that of a co-active, reciprocal, functional, first-among-equals, mentoring collaboration in the pursuit of group tasks. What kind of helping process was it that emerged from all this?

On the Nature of Helping

The legacy of group work, like that of many of the helping profes-sions, lies more in its accumulated experience and its sense of social purpose than in its understanding of its own technical skills. Towley commented on this at about the time when group work was merging its identity with that of the social work profession:

> This specialized field is rich in democratic concepts; it has a wealth of examples; but in professionally unique concepts, "method the-ory," it has been curiously poor. . . . It is possible that no social or economic class in a community is beyond profiting from what goes on under the name of a "group experience." But it is difficult for a social group worker to communicate how and why this near-miracle happens, except to another group worker.[60]

It was true; but from their "wealth of examples"–that is, the social history of their experiences with people–it is possible to bring into clearer focus some of the action implications of what the group workers thought about their purpose, knowledge, professional relationships, and the rest. Given these conceptions, and given the demands of the settings in which they worked, they were compelled to fashion certain kinds of working skills. Whether or not they were always equal to these de-

mands–early records leave some doubts on that score–the group workers nevertheless developed certain perspectives on the helping process
that were unique to their calling.

First, since the worker found himself located inside the group members' sphere of activity–a part of their play, their talk, and their transactions–his comments had to be made not as a detached observer and
interpreter but as an active participant with his own functional stake in
the proceedings. The concept of "intervention," although it would later
become fashionable, was essentially inappropriate since one does not
"intervene" in a system from the inside; it is a contradiction in terms.
Within the system, the worker's function was to provide the skills with
which to mediate the transactions between each individual and the
group, reinforcing the energies with which they reached out to each
other. In this position, two major, concurrent tasks are faced: on the one
hand, to help each member come to grips with the worker's authority
and use it to the member's own advantage; while at the same time, to
help members use each other in the collective effort. Later, Bennis and
Shepard and others would teach them more about these processes of *authority* and *intimacy*, how they operated, and the connections between
the two.[61] But whether or not they understood exactly what was happening, group workers' skills were fashioned by such demands, as were
their conceptions of the helping process in action.

Second, since the workings of groups made them often restless and
mobile, group work skills were at the outset less tuned to introspection
and the pursuit of insight than to the advancement of action. Their early
interest in non-verbal, extra-logical forms of communication had
helped them develop proficiency in many of the expressive phenomena–phantasy, play, drama, music, travelling, and the rest; it is only recently that formal courses in these "program" subjects have been
dropped from the graduate school curricula. What remains, however, is
the sensitivity to the language of action, and the awareness that talk and
action are not antithetical, the former serious and the latter trivial and
distracting, but different, often simultaneous, aspects of the communication between worker and clients.

Third, it was not possible for the worker to maintain an orderly and
logical progression of ideas when constantly being called upon to react
quickly in the press of events. The agenda was often controlled by impulse and feeling, and the worker had to develop the ability to make
quick connections and find underlying themes, protecting professional
purposes even while moving spontaneously into the action. The sight of
a worker sitting wrapped in thought while those around him were feel-

ing and acting was not calculated to inspire confidence in the interest and empathy of professional help. It was not possible for a worker successfully to urge freedom and openness on one's members while serving as a model of caution and circumspection. It called for considerable risking on the worker's part; but risking, after all, was a major ingredient in the client's prescription, and it was a poor sort of authority that gave the message to the client to "do as I say, not as I do."

Finally, since the members' main source of enjoyment and profit came from their ability to show their strengths with others, the group workers had to develop the skills with which to help the members find those strengths and use them in the group. The workers' efforts were primitive at first, relying heavily on urging and exhortation. Later, taught by Alfred Adler, Carl Rogers, and the ego psychologists, they fashioned more sophisticated techniques to mobilize client strength: partializing difficult issues; reaching for real feelings; using role-playing to help translate feelings into action; turning members toward each other for support and reality-testing; reaching for ideas that were hard to express publicly; and connecting private troubles with group concerns.

One could explore many more aspects of the group work gestalt that emerged from the need to do a helping job within a setting that, because it was social, public, and on the clients' home ground, made unusual demands upon the worker. This is not to say that the helping process in group work was *sui generis*, or totally different from other approaches; indeed the point of this paper is that it was only a special manifestation of social work in action. But, over and above the similarities, group work's special character lay in the fact that its experience brought into focus certain phenomena that are less easily seen when the work is private, one-on-one, and under the worker's almost total control.

Toward an Expanded Paradigm

The old settlement idea of the helping relationship as a shared experience meant that residents and neighbors, workers and group members, were on a voyage of discovery, affecting each other's lives, tied together with a common bond, fulfilling each one's own special purposes in the process. The idea was drawn from the very air of Victorian society; it was class-dominated, idealistic, and amateurish in many ways. But its deeper truth lay in its vision of a relationship in which the qualities of leadership were expressed in the joys of human collaboration, rather than in the action of the knower on the naive, the strong on the weak, the expert on the uninitiated. As I have indicated, the intimacy of worker and members created the need to guard one's function carefully, lest it be lost in the close exchange. But the opposite view–detached, "objective," and often identified as more *truly* professional–raises a more serious problem; the distance between worker and client is then so large, and the worker's position on the periphery of the system so secure, that there is no longer any risk at all, and the worker is too safe to worry about it. The group worker's emotional involvement, and tenuous control of the situation, felt dangerous but it was often salutary. Caseworkers who have moved into service with groups have experienced this sense of danger as the feeling, "there are so many of them and only one of me!"[62] They have found that

> . . . the group leadership role demands that the worker give up much of the interview control to which she has, often unconsciously, become accustomed. Caseworkers have often told me that they had never realized how rigidly they controlled the client-worker interaction until they began to function as group workers, where changes of subject could be effected by anyone in the group, where people often turned to each other rather than to the worker for reinforcement and support, where clients could verify each other's "wrong" ideas, where mutually reinforced feelings could not be turned off when they became "dangerous," and where, in short, one's faith in the client's autonomy and basic strength were put to its severest test.[63]

These are the themes of shared control, shared power, and the shared agenda, which are among those I have tried to identify in this paper. That their appearance is so disconcerting to those who first move into group service speaks well for their potential uses in helping to evolve a richer model of the helping process in social work. Each theme needs to be explored in some detail: the social self, the faith in action, the helping relationship as a reciprocal system, the shared power, the sense of immediacy, the eclecticism, the collective sources of individual strength, and even, in some respects, the didacticism that pervaded the group workers' outlook.

The ideas themselves are not new; many have in certain ways been accepted over the years. But they are easy to lose sight of, in a model of practice–perhaps it is the coveted medical model–of a unilateral power exercised over an objectified, inert, malleable client. For example, the definition of the self as a social creation, culturally formed and culturally modifiable, is well ensconced in today's scientific atmosphere; but it is hard to keep before us in the paradigm of the client as a broken object who comes to be repaired by an agent of change who operates single-handedly on self-contained, privately-owned personalities.

As to what it is that does help people change in their own chosen direction,[64] that question will be with us for a long time. The group workers' experience told them that there was something in the nature of *doing*, and particularly collective doing, that helped people find new ways of looking at themselves and the world around them. Many, like Neva Boyd, suspected verbal and logical explanations that went under the name of "insight," but seemed to produce more "aha"s than lasting changes in problem-solving behavior. And it was Kierkegaard, a generation before Freud, who said that "truth exists for the individual only as he himself produces it in action."[65] Ultimately, of course, the answer will lie not in pitting action against insight, but in finding the connections between the two, and the techniques with which to distinguish real understanding from verbal games, and meaningful action from a mechanical behaviorism.

And so it would go: there is obviously a great deal more to be done with these issues than can be attempted here. The major threads are reciprocal, systemic, existential, and would lead us back into studies that might rescue these constructs from their stereotypes and translate them back into their implications for practice, both one-to-one and one-to-group. For the present, this brief analysis may help bring their roots in the group work experience back into view and lead the profession forward in the process of locating the traditions that indeed make up the profession.

FOOTNOTES AND REFERENCES

1. Kathleen Woodroofe, *From Charity to Social Work* (Toronto: University of Toronto Press, 1962), p. 46.

2. Robert H. Bremner, *American Philanthropy* (Chicago: The University of Chicago Press, 1960), pp. 95 ff.

3. American Association of Social Workers, *Social Case Work, Generic and Specific: An Outline: A Report of the Milford Conference*, 1929, 92 pages.

4. "The TIAC Report: Principles, Proposals and Issues in Inter-Association Cooperation," *Social Work Journal*, Vol. 32, No. 3 (July 1951), pp. 112-57. Entire issue on the subject.

5. Melvin A. Glasser. "The Story of the Movement for a Single Professional Association." *Social Work Journal*, Vol. 36, No. 3 (July 1955), pp. 115-22.

6. Talcott Parsons, "A Sociologist Looks at the Legal Profession," in *Essays in Sociological Theory* (Glencoe. Ill.: The Free Press. 1954, Rev. Ed.), p. 372.

7. *See*, for example: Harriet M. Burden, "Toward Clarification and Improvement of Social Work Practice," *Social Work*, Vol. 3, No. 2 (April 1958), pp. 3-9. *See also*: "The Generic-Specific Concept in Social Work Education and Practice," in Alfred J. Kahn (ed.), *Issues in American Social Work* (New York: Columbia University Press, 1959), pp. 159-90.

8. William E. Gordon, "A Critique of the Working Definition," *Social Work*, Vol. 7, No. 4 (October 1962), pp. 3-13.

9. For an earlier historical effort of my own, *see:* William Schwartz, "Group Work and the Social Scene." in Alfred E. Kahn (ed.), *Issues in American Social Work* (New York: Columbia University Press, 1959), pp. 110-37.

10. Henrietta Barnett, *Canon Barnett, His Life, Work, and Friends, By His Wife* (Boston and New York: Houghton Mifflin Company, 1919, 2 Volumes), Vol. I, pp. 27 ff.

11. Mary E. Richmond, *Social Diagnosis* (New York: Russell Sage Foundation, 1917).

12. Grace L. Coyle, *Social Process in Organized Groups* (New York: Richard R. Smith, 1930).

13. Henrietta Barnett, op. cit., p. 184.

14. *See*: Mrs. Glendower Evans, "Scientific Charity," *Proceedings of the National Conference of Charities and Correction, 1889* (Boston: Geo. H. Ellis. 1889), pp. 24-35.

15. *See*: William Schwartz, "Camping," *Social Work Year Book, 1960* (New York: National Association of Social Workers, 1960), pp. 112-17.

16. Margaretta Williamson, *The Social Worker in Group Work* (New York and London: Harper, 1929), p. 17.

17. William Heard Kilpatrick, *Group Education for a Democracy* (New York: Association Press, 1940), p. vii.

18. Grace Coyle, "On Becoming Professional," in *Toward Professional Standards* (New York: American Association of Group Workers, 1947), pp. 17-18.

19. Schwartz, "Group Work and the Social Scene," op. cit., p. 123.

20. For the distinction between the "priests," who minister to the needy without judging them, and the "prophets," who thunder and hold up standards to follow, *see*: Clarke A. Chambers, "An Historical Perspective on Political Action vs. Individualized Treatment," in *Current Issues in Social Work Seen in Historical Perspective* (New York: Council on Social Work Education, 1962), p. 54.

21. Quoted in Clarke A. Chambers, *Seedtime of Reform: American Social Service and Social Action, 1918-1933* (Minneapolis: University of Minnesota Press, 1963), p. 150.

22. Ibid., p. 149.

23. Eduard C. Lindeman, "Group Work and Democracy—A Philosophical Note." reprinted in Albert S. Alissi (ed.), *Perspectives on Small Group Work Practice* (New York: The Free Press, 1980), p. 81. Originally published in 1939.

24. Jane Addams, *Twenty Years at Hull House* (New York: The New American Library, A Signet Classic, 1960), p. 97. First published in 1910.

25. Henrietta Barnett, *Canon Barnett, His Life, Work, and Friends. . . .*, op. cit., p. 110.

26. Henrietta Barnett, "Principles of Recreation," in Canon and Mrs. S. A. Barnett, *Towards Social Reform* (New York: The Macmillan Company, 1909), p. 289.

27. Eduard C. Lindeman, "Organization and Technique for Rural Recreation," *Proceedings of the National Conference of Social Work* (Chicago: University of Chicago Press, 1920), p. 321.

28. Henrietta Barnett, *Canon Barnett, His Life, Work, and Friends. . . .*, op. cit., p. 115.

29. Canon Barnett, "'Settlements' or 'Missions,'" in Canon and Mrs. S. A. Barnett, op. cit., p. 273.

30. Ibid., pp. 271-88.

31. Charles Horton Cooley, *Social Organization: A Study of the Larger Mind* (New York: Schocken Books, 1962), p. 23, First published in 1909, by Charles Scribner's Sons.

32. Ibid., p. 29. Emphasis in original.

33. Ibid., p. 23.

34. James Mark Baldwin, *The Individual and Society* (Boston: Richard G. Badger, The Gorham Press, 1911), p. 16.

35. P. Kropotkin, *Mutual Aid, A Factor of Evolution* (New York: Alfred A. Knopf, 1925).

36. John Dewey, *Human Nature and Conduct* (New York: Random House, 1922).

37. George Herbert Mead, *Mind, Self and Society* (Chicago: University of Chicago Press, 1934).

38 Muzafer Sherif, *The Psychology of Social Norms* (New York: Harper, 1936).

39. Kurt Lewin, "Conduct, Knowledge, and Acceptance of New Values," in *Resolving Social Conflicts: Selected Papers on Group Dynamics* (New York: Harper, 1948), pp. 56-68.

40. Baldwin, op. cit., p. 16.

41. Mary Parker Follett, "Constructive Conflict," in Henry C. Metcalf and L. Urwick (eds.), *Dynamic Administration: The Collected Papers of Mary Parker Follett* (New York and London: Harper, 1940), p. 45. Paper first published in 1926.

42. Martin Buber, *I and Thou* (New York: Charles Scribner's Sons, 1958).

43. Neva L. Boyd, "The Social Education of Youth Through Recreation: The Value of Play in Education," in Paul Simon (ed.), *Play and Game Theory in Group Work: A Collection of Papers by Neva Leona Boyd* (Chicago: The Jane Addams Graduate School of Social Work at the University of Illinois at Chicago Circle, 1971), p. 43. Paper written in 1924.

44. Neva L. Boyd, "Social Group Work: A Definition with a Methodological Note," in Paul Simon (ed.), op. cit., p. 149. Paper written in 1937.

45. Ibid.

46. LeRoy E. Bowman, "Dictatorship, Democracy, and Group Work in America," *Proceedings of the National Conference of Social Work* (Chicago: University of Chicago Press, 1935), p. 385.

47. Virginia P. Robinson, "The Dynamics of Supervision under Functional Controls," in *The Development of a Professional Self. Teaching and Learning in Professional Helping Processes, Selected Writings, 1930-1968* (New York: AMS Press, 1978), p. 254. Article first published in 1948.

48. Grace Longwell Coyle, *Group Work with American Youth: A Guide to the Practice of Leadership* (New York: Harper, 1948), p. 32.

49. LeRoy Bowman, op. cit., p. 383.

50. For a discussion of this "symbiotic" relationship between the individual and his group, *see*: William Schwartz, "The Social Worker in the Group," *The Social Welfare Forum, 1961* (New York and London: Columbia University Press, 1961), pp. 156 ff.

51. For a discussion of the social work function in regard to the needs of the one and the many, *see*: William Schwartz, "Private Troubles and Public Issues: One Social Work Job or Two?" *The Social Welfare Forum, 1969* (New York and London: Columbia University Press, 1969), pp. 22-43.

52. Henrietta Barnett, *Canon Barnett, His Life, Work, and Friends. . . .* op. cit., p. 169.

53. Mrs. Glendower Evans, op, cit., p. 25.

54. Sigmund Freud, "The Dynamics of the Transference," (1912), *Collected Papers* (London: The Hogarth Press and The Institute of Psycho-Analysis, 1950, 5 Volumes), Vol. II, pp. 312-22.

55. Ibid., p. 318.

56. Sigmund Freud, "Recommendations for Physicians on the Psycho-Analytic Method of Treatment," (1912) *Collected Papers* (London. The Hogarth Press and The Institute of Psycho-Analysis, 1950, 5 Volumes), Vol. II, p. 331.

57. LeRoy Bowman, op. cit., pp. 385-6.

58. Mary Parker Follett, "Some Discrepancies in Leadership Theory and Practice," in Metcalf and Urwick (egos, op. cit., p. 272). Emphasis in original. Article first published in 1928.

59. Grace Longwell Coyle, *Group Work With American Youth . . . ,* op. cit., p. 216.

60. Frank J. Bruno (with chapters by Louis Towley), *Trends in Social Work, 1874-1956* (New York: Columbia University Press, 1957), p. 422.

61. Warren G. Bennis & H. A. Shepard, "A Theory of Group Development," *Human Relations*, Vol. 9 (1956), pp. 415-37.

62. William Schwartz, "Discussion of Three Papers on the Group Method with Clients, Foster Families, and Adoptive Families," *Child Welfare*, Vol. 45, No. 10 (December 1966), p. 572.

63. Ibid., p. 575.

64. *See*, for example: Allen Wheelis, "How People Change," *Commentary* (May 1969), pp. 56-66.

65. Quoted in Rollo May, "The Emergence of Existential Psychology," in Rollo May, (ed.), *Existential Psychology* (New York: Random House, 1961), p. 12.

Building Mutual Support in Groups

Alex Gitterman

SUMMARY. The concept of support is frequently referred to in the groupwork literature but is relatively underdeveloped and unspecified. This paper partializes the concept of support and identifies and illustrates specific professional behaviors which are essential to the building of support in a group. *[Article copies available for a fee from The Haworth Document Delivery Service: 1-800-HAWORTH. E-mail address: <docdelivery@haworthpress.com> Website: <http://www.HaworthPress.com> © 2005 by The Haworth Press, Inc. All rights reserved.]*

Support is integral to the group modality. It provides a major rationale for the provision of group services. In fact, such services are often referred to as "support groups." While the concept is frequently referred to in the literature, it is rarely defined and specified.[1] The notion of support is so central to our practice, that we have, perhaps unjustifiably, assumed a common understanding about it and dealt with it as if it were too self-evident and obvious to clarify and specify. The notion of peer support has consequently remained somewhat ambiguous, and undefined. For similar and more complex reasons, the professional behaviors and actual processes of building mutual support in a group have

Alex Gitterman, EdD, is Professor, Columbia University School of Social Work.

This paper is based upon a presentation at the Center for Groupwork Studies Annual Symposium, Berry University, 1987.

This article was originally published in *Social Work with Groups*, Vol. 12 (2) © 1989 by The Haworth Press, Inc.

[Haworth co-indexing entry note]: "Building Mutual Support in Groups." Gitterman, Alex. Co-published simultaneously in *Social Work with Groups* (The Haworth Press, Inc.) Vol. 28, No. 3/4, 2005, pp. 91-106; and: *A Quarter Century of Classics (1978-2004): Capturing the Theory, Practice, and Spirit of Social Work with Groups* (ed: Andrew Malekoff, and Roselle Kurland) The Haworth Press, Inc., 2005, pp. 91-106. Single or multiple copies of this article are available for a fee from The Haworth Document Delivery Service [1-800-HAWORTH, 9:00 a.m. - 5:00 p.m. (EST). E-mail address: docdelivery@haworthpress.com].

Available online at http://www.haworthpress.com/web/SWG
© 2005 by The Haworth Press, Inc. All rights reserved.
doi:10.1300/J009v28n03_07

also remained relatively underdeveloped and unspecified. The purpose of this paper, therefore, is to partialize the concept of support and to identify and illustrate specific professional behaviors which are essential to the processes of building support in a group.

GROUP SUPPORT

Support can be metaphorically compared to providing the function to a group that energy provides to machinery. As members begin to feel supported by and in the group, they are more likely to share their concerns and experiences and take a chance on becoming involved with each other, and thus accomplish the purpose of the group. While they initially may share safe and less threatening issues, they are actually testing each others's and the worker's genuineness and competence. As members experience continuing support, they are likely to risk more personal, even taboo concerns. This process itself helps members to experience their concerns and problems as being less private and deviant. This process reduces isolation, "de-pathologises" problems and diminishes stigma. As members reach out to each other, they experience a variety of helping relationships and become increasingly invested in each other and in participating in interpersonal processes. Mutual support encourages members to struggle, to offer and receive help from each other rather than leaving that job primarily to the worker. Since group members have had common experiences and problems, they are often receptive to each others' views, suggestions and challenges. Without support (like machines without energy), groups are likely to lose their drive and momentum.

For members to experience and to be experienced by others as supportive, they have to be able to demonstrate and convey to each other specific kinds of behaviors. *Acceptance* is one example. To accept another requires an ability to be emotionally and cognitively with another person. This is demonstrated by such actions as conveying to another their worth, demonstrating care and interest, and offering suggestions without value judgements and moral lectures.[2] Offering *hope* is another behavior which demonstrates support. When members experience a sense that situations can change, become easier or less stressful, they are more likely than otherwise to invest themselves in the group. Being helped to feel that one has one's own as well as the group's collective resources to make things different and better are powerful incentives to undertaking new problem solving strategies and behaviors. Finally, support is provided and experienced through tangible behaviors of helping each other to learn the actual skills of competently managing one's feelings and developing pertinent problem-solving strategies. Group members provide support by helping each other to manage overwhelming feelings of anxiety, or devastating pain from loss and isolation, or incapacitating self-doubts and insecurities. When members deny or rationalize, others may provide support by eliciting such feelings as anxiety or dissatisfaction with the status quo. Beyond managing feelings, effective coping requires the competence to solve problems. Being supportive is helping members learn how to help each other to solve their difficulties.[3]

FORMING MUTUAL SUPPORT GROUPS

In forming a mutual support group, the first professional task is to identify a clear purpose. Common needs, concerns or interests provide the foundation for support. The worker starts with a clear idea about group purpose, translating commonalty into specific operational tasks. Groups can be formed around typical life stresses, i.e., problems-in-living that people experience. Life transitional networking includes forming groups to deal with such common issues and concerns as: particular developmental struggles (learning disabled adolescents, young adult diabetics); difficult life statuses (siblings of retarded youngsters, homeless adults, renal dialysis patients, separating and divorcing parents); desired and undesired life changes (school transitions, marriage, parenthood, retirement, immigration, admission and discharge from institutions) and crisis events (pre or post surgery, chronic or acute illness, physical trauma and assault, loss of loved one). Environmental networking includes forming groups to deal with such common issues and concerns as: isolated elderly, parents of retarded children, problems within an organization (institutional food, welfare rights, tenants association) and consumer involvement within an agency (planning committee, advisory group, leadership council). Interpersonal networking includes forming groups to deal with common interpersonal issues and concerns experienced within natural units (couples, multi-family groups) and working with existing collectivities (patients on wards, children in residential cottages and students in a classroom). The problems in living formulation provides a guideline for clustering people at risk of social and emotional isolation.[4]

Group composition, another professional task, has a profound influence upon interpersonal processes. For the development of optimal mutual support, group members require both the stability from compositional homogeneity and the diversity from compositional heterogeneity. Ideally, both should be present. In composing a group for pregnant adolescents, for example, the worker considers the following factors: common concerns about "birthing"; relationship with parents, boyfriends, peers, school representatives; future plans for babies, etc. The worker also considers the relative advantages and disadvantages of commonalty and differences in such other factors as age, first pregnancy, religion, ethnicity, stage of pregnancy, etc. As a rule, members usually benefit from diversity when common interests and concerns are experienced intensively. Thus, for example, a group formed to help members cope with cancer is likely to be able to use compositional diversity more effectively than a group formed for a more general and ambiguous purpose of helping with adolescence. In the latter group, compositional differences are likely to result in interpersonal conflict and squabble. In contrast, the common situations of cancer patients (i.e., set of common fears and expectations) is such a powerful commonalty that it is able to incorporate individual differences in background and personality. The worker must assume responsibility for group composition. To relinquish this responsibility to someone else, e.g., a teacher in a secondary setting may result in a group of only acting-out children, or, if to a nurse, a group composed of diabetics with severely mixed symptomatology (i.e., early and amputation stages). Such combinations do not encourage mutual support and end in either conflict or despair or both.[5] A client poignantly describes the experience of being "different" in a group:

> My previous social worker referred me to a group at a mental health clinic. She told me it would give me something to do and people other than my children to talk to. Then I found out it was a group for recently released hospital patients many of whom were still psychotic. They talked to themselves and sometimes lost sight of reality for moments. I was frightened by them, and also upset that I was placed in a group with them. Look, I know I'm nuts, but I'm not that nuts. Maybe sometime I will be, but let me get there in my own time. When I have a nervous breakdown, I want it to be my very own and not taught to me by members of my therapy group.[6]

Some groups tend to be long-term and open-ended with departing members replaced by new members. When a common membership core remains intact, these groups provide long lasting emotional support, social contact and instrumental assistance. When membership fluctuates, these groups tend to develop two chronic problems: (1) loss of original sense of purpose and vitality and (2) members remain stuck in an early stage of group development. In contrast, the time boundary in planned short-term and time-limited groups helps members focus quickly, maintain purpose, direction and a sense of urgency. Other time considerations are frequency and duration of each meeting. Children and cognitively emotionally impaired adults, for examples, are both responsive to more frequent and shorter sessions. Thus, structuring temporal arrangements is another professional task useful in the development of mutual support.

BEGINNING A MUTUAL SUPPORT GROUP

Shared definition of concerns or problems, explicit mutual agreement about goals, and about respective roles engages members' motivation and cognition. It also develops reciprocal accountability and provides focus to the work.[7] In offering a group service, the worker's primary task is to capture the members' perception of their life situation, maintaining an ethical balance between active outreach and respect for a person's right to refuse service. With the person upon whom group service is mandated, the worker's primary obligation is to acknowledge and deal directly with the fact of imposition of service. Further, the task is to locate areas of discomfort (usually located in the environment) and specify the nature of the mandate and possible sanctions for noncooperation. These initial entry strategies are essential to the development of mutual support and are enhanced by several core contracting skills, the most important of which include:

1. *Presenting the agency's group service in clear and concrete terms*: Members require a clear understanding about the groups' purpose to evaluate appropriateness and suitability. Informed members are less likely to fear hidden agenda and, more likely to be receptive to an offer of help.

2. *Identifying group members' potential perceptions of their needs, problems or interests*: There are potentially differing perceptions between the agency, the worker and group members. Children, for example, referred by a teacher for being "troublemakers" may feel that they

are not liked and are being picked on. Similarly, mentally retarded young adults may not appreciate being referred to as "mentally retarded," and may be more responsive to a description of the effect of their common status on their lives, e.g., being teased for being slow and treated like a child. These sensitivities encourage mutually supportive behaviors.

3. *Identifying professional role and its boundaries*: Group members need to know that they are meeting with a social worker and have some idea about what social workers do. (To the query of "what does your father do?" a colleague's younger child responded, "He goes to meetings and helps people.") Children in a school group, for example, will use their teachers as role models for expected adult behaviors. With these expectations, mutual support would be inhibited.

4. *Translating members' needs into priorities*: Members' statement of need and an agency's offer of service do not in themselves represent a mutual agreement until members and worker have reached an explicit understanding about their particular foci and priorities. Translating needs into tasks and setting priorities offers worker and members a common frame of reference. Several guidelines are useful in developing priorities: (1) identification of the most pressing and stressful issues in members' lives. Paying attention to members' *vulnerabilities* provides the worker with critical points of entry into their lives; (2) avoidance of mobilizing individual member's and the group's systems of defenses. By selecting concerns which will initially mobilize least *resistance*, the worker takes care to begin with the members' definition and perceptions of their problems. When parents, for example, initially define their children as the "problem," redefining the problem as a marital one is very apt to mobilize defensiveness and withdrawal and (3) selection of tasks which provide the opportunity for positive outcomes. *Success* is a powerful motivator for involvement and mutual support.

These skills have to be employed flexibly, depending upon members' cognitive style, level of physical, emotional and social functioning, their backgrounds and the agency context.

BUILDING MUTUAL SUPPORT

As the work begins, the worker's authority, function and boundaries receive particular attention. And this provides the worker with still another task–to deal with a testing process through which members will develop and reinforce mutual support and alliances as they struggle to figure out where the worker belongs in the interpersonal system. A few years ago the author worked with a group of high school girls. At our third meeting, a member with the support of others expressed their discomfort by asking him to share a happy and painful life experience. At that moment, the group coalesced to test his willingness to "belong" to the group. The members responded to his sharing a happy experience as well as a painful loss, by sharing their own losses (death of a parent, divorce, etc.), and so began some moving, focused and intense work. Another example is a social work student who was assigned to a group of recently released mental patients who had been meeting for a year:

> I stated that I understood this patient group had been meeting for about a year. Mrs. Bates interrupted by saying, "I don't like being called a patient." I asked her, "how come." Mrs. Bates suggested in effect that "patient" connoted sickness. I asked the other group members how they felt about it. Mrs. Charles agreed she did not like to be classified as a patient either. Mr. Anthony asked her what she wanted to be called. Mrs. Charles paused thoughtfully for a moment and said she would like to be called a "client." I asked the rest of the group for their reactions. Mrs. Bates said that was alright, but she would just like to be called a "member." The group responded positively to this, saying that they liked "member" better. I said that since I was new to the group and they had been *members* for some time, could they bring me up-to-date on the how the group began, what they talked about, dealt with and so on.

While the members may be "crazy," they certainly are not "stupid." They make an extremely sophisticated point about wanting to be treated with respect rather than being "treated." The group members here challenge the worker whose openness encourages the elaboration of mutual support. If she had turned their concerns into manifestations of psychological problems or had not treated the content with the seriousness and respect needed, members might have withdrawn or engaged in mutually exploitative behavior.

To build a mutual support system, the worker helps group members to develop a sense of commonalty and integration. To facilitate achievement of this essential group task, requires of the worker particular skills.

1. *Directing members' transactions to each other*: In the early stages of work with groups, members usually communicate through the worker. Like a "telephone switchboard operator" arranging a "conference call,"

the worker attempts to help members to talk directly to each other. In so doing, the worker encourages the development of mutual support.

2. *Inviting members to build on each other's contributions*: People often talk at each other rather than to each other. By linking a member's comment to those of others–"Bill's idea is very close to George's, what do the rest of you think about their idea?"–the worker encourages members to become involved with each other and to facilitate mutual support.

3. *Reinforcing mutual support and assistance norms*: Out of their individual beliefs, knowledge and value orientations, group members develop collective norms regarding rights and responsibilities, modes of work, and styles of relating and communicating. In some groups, members learn to compete with, withdraw from, and/or exploit each other. To mitigate these maladaptive norms, the worker encourages and reinforces cooperative mutual support norms. This is accomplished by modeling, teaching and crediting their expression, saying, "I hope you feel great about how you solved this problem–no one yelled, teased, threatened, rather you helped each other" reinforces and encourages mutual support.

4. *Examining group sanctions*: Shared beliefs about style and quality of interactions and verbal and physical expression of thoughts and feelings are enforced by explicit and implicit means. These include disapproval and stronger sanctions, interpersonal punishment ranging from mild rebukes and teasing to more extreme responses as scapegoating and ostracism. Clear and flexible sanctions encourage mutual support, ambiguous and rigid ones tend to factionalize members. By helping members to examine their patterns for expression of approval and disapproval, the worker attempts to help them to develop clearer behavioral guidelines and greater acceptance. When members are clear about what behaviors are preferred, permitted, proscribed and prohibited, they are likely to be less anxious and more available to each other.

5. *Encouraging collective action and activities*: Members need opportunities to act in their collective interests and participate in mutually satisfying activities. Action and activities play crucial roles in development and learning, both across the life cycle, and in coping and adaptation. They require planning and decision making, interaction and communication, specification of roles and tasks, and, frequently, negotiating the social and physical environment. By encouraging collective activities and by experiencing collective successes, the group becomes a source of mutual support and satisfaction. For a group of regressed schizophrenics, the activity of preparing coffee, for example, comfortably structures interaction and brings members closer together. To experience success,

the worker and group members must determine their readiness and motivation to undertake the collective action or activity.

6. *Clarifying members tasks and role responsibilities*: In order to undertake collective action and activities, a worker needs to help members to develop a division of labor. A group, for example, planning a camping trip has to specify the essential tasks (purchase of food and supplies, cooking of meals, setting up tents, etc.) and allocate specific responsibility for completion of the tasks ("Let's agree on what chores have to be done during the week, decide who is doing what and talk about what changes might help"). Specification of tasks and role assignment (i.e., a division of labor) facilitates mutual support and interpersonal integration and reduces conflict and stress.

7. *Structuring collective decision making*: In some groups, members experience difficulty in making group decisions, and require help with learning such processes as achieving consensus and compromise. These processes though often caught also have to be taught. The author, for example, worked with a group of disadvantaged older adolescent boys who were unable to plan, to problem solve or even to sustain a simple, focussed discussion. A member's comment would be immediately punctuated by another member's sneer or jeer about a girlfriend, mother, and so on. Chaos invariably followed! Since they had neither experienced nor learned the value of collaborative decision making, a structure was provided to facilitate collaborative processes. An interactional sequence was developed with them to use in planning any program or making any decision: (1) in a round robin fashion each member presented one idea at a time which was recorded on a large master list. The round robin continued until all members ideas were expressed (during this step no comments or alternative suggestions were allowed); (2) discussion about each alternative was limited to clarification and identification of potential problems; (3) after duplicate ideas were eliminated and impractical alternatives voluntarily withdrawn, the group voted for the preferred plan or decision. The prescribed sequence provided a structure for decision making and eliminated disabling criticisms and harshness. And as members learned to listen to each other, interpersonal support and competence replaced interpersonal exploitation and inadequacy.

8. *Identifying and focusing on salient group themes*: In working with groups, the worker confronts simultaneous and competing cues. At times the theme is evident and relatively easy to identify (adoptive youngsters asking questions about their natural parents). Other times, the group theme is more elusive and expressed in disparate behaviors

and responses (group of youngsters differentially coping with group termination). To be helpful, the worker searches for, identifies and focuses on common integrating themes ("I sense you are all very curious about your biological parents . . ." or "Everybody is reacting to the group's ending . . . John, you're running in and out of the room; Bill, you have stopped talking to me; Jack, you have laid your head down and closed your eyes; and I am acting like the group is not ending in two weeks . . ."). By identifying and focusing on the common salient themes, the worker provides the "glue" to bind members together and help each other with mutual concerns and issues.

Through the skills discussed in this section, the worker helps to integrate members by developing and elaborating common themes and structures which call forth mutual support. These themes and structures strengthen collective functioning and are essential to a system of support. While essential, however, they are not sufficient. To develop a mutual support system, the worker also has to help each group member to negotiate his/her individual needs for being different and separate. Developing a satisfactory balance between the demands for integration and individuation, requires of the worker particular and specific skills.

9. *Reaching for discrepant perceptions and opinions*: A worker has to be extremely careful about encouraging a premature consensus and stifling divergent perceptions and opinions. By inviting individual members to disagree, to have differing opinions and perceptions ("John, I sense you don't fully agree–I'm very interested in your thoughts"), the worker encourages expression of individual differences. A collectivity is only as strong as its ability to allow and tolerate differences. Members can only be supportive of each other, if they feel sufficient comfort to state their thoughts and feelings openly.

10. *Inviting and "chasing" individual members to participate*: Due to the transactional fit between group composition and individual member attributes, some members may experience difficulty in participating and may either withdraw, engage in parallel activities or act-out. At times, these behaviors are simply situational or episodic; while other times, they represent long established patterns. With caring and support, the worker invites the participation of the "outside" member. Often, more than one invitation is necessary; interest and caring are demonstrated through several invitations–"Billy, Debby is most worried about what to expect in high school, what's mostly on your mind?" By active inviting and chasing of individual member's participation, the worker conveys and models the importance of each member in the group.

11. *Creating emotional and physical space for individual members*: Group members have diverse needs for intimacy and distance, group activity and individual solitude, and group unity and individual distinctiveness. Some members require more separateness and space than do others. The worker attempts to help group members struggle to achieve a comfortable balance, identifying and supporting a member's need for greater space–"I think John is saying he needs a little more time before he is ready to talk . . ."

As members feel more comfortable and less threatened, they become more invested with each other. When their individual styles and rhythms are respected and valued, they become willing to take chances and to lower their defenses. Thus, for the worker, a critical professional task is to assure that individual needs are balanced with group needs.

OBSTACLES TO MUTUAL SUPPORT

In coping with life transitions, environments and internal group processes, members encounter interpersonal obstacles. These obstacles are expressed in maladaptive communication and relationship patterns. Stress is generated in the system, hindering mutual support. Withdrawal, factionalism, alliances and scapegoating are illustrative of these maladaptive patterns. While maladaptive for most members, these patterned behaviors also serve a latent need for maintaining group functioning. Scapegoating, for example, may stave off difficulties in the group while promoting it in the scapegoated member.[8] After a while these patterns may well become fixed and potential change resisted. To mitigate these maladaptive patterns, the worker uses various direct as well as indirect professional skills.

1. *Identifying maladaptive patterns*: Members are often unaware of their transactional patterns. Identifying a maladaptive pattern observing that "I've noticed every time someone introduces a painful and scary concern like graduating, getting drunk, girlfriends cheating, someone picks on John and our focus changes . . ." is often a first step to consciousness raising. As the pattern repeats itself, the worker can reflect on prior interventions ("O.K., here we go again, it's happening right now, Bill, you just started in on John when we began to talk about your father's drinking . . .). The worker can also encourage members to either give up a pattern even if slowly by suggesting, "Come on let's not start on John, Bill what happened the last time your father came home

drunk . . ." or examining the pattern directly–"Let's talk about what's happening right now."

2. *Challenging collective resistance*: Often, group members can not readily accept a worker's identification of maladaptive transactional patterns. To give up entrenched patterns is far from easy. Avoiding conflict, painful material, intimacy and threatening changes or escaping into an "illusion of work" may be initially an easier and understandable defense. For mutual support to serve the group's purpose, however, the worker has to attend to the dysfunctional patterns, hold members to their contract and to the work, "Everybody is fuming but nobody is talking, what's going on? . . . this silence won't solve any problems, what's happening? . . . Bull, it's not O.K., you are all very upset, what happened?" Such professional directness and persistence convey strength and genuine caring, which can release members' energies to deal with group tasks and with each other. Challenging dysfunctional patterns may induce a crisis which can loosen entrenched processes and structures to allow communication and relational patterns to improve.

3. *Inviting and sustaining group conflict*: When anger is suppressed or denied, communication is thwarted and mutual support wanes. The worker invites and sustains the expression of these feelings, reactions and associated content as in "I would like each one of you to put your silence into words, what's annoying you about . . . ?" By inviting negative feelings and thoughts, the worker conveys interest and respect for each member and faith in their ability to communicate and work on interpersonal issues. And by overcoming them, mutual support is enhanced.

4. *Reaching for discrepant perceptions and disagreements*: Members often need assistance and encouragement to express their discrepant perceptions and disagreements–"Phyllis, you disagree with the idea of getting a lawyer who will take a husband to 'the cleaners?'" By helping members to elaborate their opinions and explore differences and disagreements, the worker reaches for open and honest exchanges and consequently deepens the work.

5. *Establishing protective ground rules*: If members are to feel sufficiently comfortable to participate in discussion of disagreements and conflicts, they need a secure atmosphere in which differences can be examined without fear of recrimination. Thus, the worker has to establish ground rules which protect and facilitate open and direct conversations. Explicit rules barring use of physical violence, verbal abuse or threat have to be established. Such rules provide structural and normative supports for the weaker, lower status member. The worker insistently en-

courages and, even, demands that members abide by the agreed upon rules.

6. *Searching for and identifying common definitions and perceptions*: As members consider their differences, the worker listens carefully for possible common definitions and perceptions. For example, an adolescent group invited their parents to a meeting to work on the conflicts between them. A critical theme emerged; the adolescents' struggle to acquire greater freedom and autonomy and the reciprocal parental struggle to maintain some control and direction over the lives of their children. In helping the arguments unfold, the worker began to search for possible common definitions and perceptions. The parents' strong stake in their children making a safe transition to young adulthood; the adolescents' stake in their parents' providing sufficient protection and direction for them. After exploring their diverse perceptions and disagreements, the worker identified the "common ground" between them. By identifying common definitions and perceptions, members are directed to one another to search for some consensus and mutual support.

7. *Lending support and crediting work*: Staying with conflict and searching for common ground requires open and direct communication. Group members need support and credit for their willingness to struggle and to risk themselves (e.g., "The important thing is that as mad as you were at each other, you were able to talk about it . . . it was hard to do, but you've done it real well!").

8. *Using indirect means to facilitate communication*: When group members are unable to discuss the interpersonal difficulties, the worker uses indirect interventions to facilitate communication. Activities, programs and nonverbal methods can encourage interpersonal involvement and mutual support.[9] Audio and videotape provides members with the opportunity to hear and see themselves in action and discuss it as the worker stops and plays back the transactions. Between sessions, assignments of tasks can be used. These may include shared activities and monitoring uncooperative behavior, to encourage improvement of communication and mutual support.

Relationship and communication obstacles are phenomena inherent in a group's life. Members usually have some ambivalence about intimacy, about being close to each other and with the worker. As members work out such issues, they become closer, supportive, and helpful to each other. Usually with the worker's encouragement and professional skills, the interpersonal tensions diminish and energies are released for the agreed upon tasks. When these obstacles are ignored or dealt with unskillfully, they become entrenched and threaten the group's existence. The worker, thus, has to have confidence in the members and in his/her abilities to deal with the maladaptive patterns. By meeting the challenge, members have the opportunity to gain greater self and collective confidence and learn about the quintessential meaning of mutual support.

CONCLUSION

The paper has attempted to clarify and specify professional tasks and skills associated with building mutual support in groups. The author hopes he has not implied that the professional tasks and skills identified and discussed are to be applied prescriptively and in a neat, logical, orderly and sequential fashion. For in a group, the worker faces an array of simultaneous themes and cues, at times perplexing and other times overwhelming. At every and any moment, the worker has to determine which ones to respond to, and which to table. There is very little time to think and strategize about the "correct" intervention.

What can the worker fall back on in these moments?

The problems-in-living formulation provides a framework which encourages greater focus and direction to practice interventions. To illustrate, a worker is trying to help a group composed of recent widows. In the fourth session, members are agitated and complain about their loneliness and isolation. Were they at this particular moment asking for help in exploring their grief and going through the mourning process (i.e., life transition)? Or were they asking for help with their sense of social isolation and in becoming more effectively connected to their support systems or possibly requesting help in acquiring new support systems (i.e., environment)? Or, finally, were they at this particular moment, indirectly complaining about the worker's and group's lack of support and obliquely requesting attention to their own internal group issues (i.e., interpersonal)? How a worker intervenes would be different depending upon an assessment about whether the help being sought was life transitional, environmental or interpersonal. The problems in living formulation may assist the worker in choosing the appropriate interventions at each moment after each session and over longer time intervals.

A small, important concluding note: The worker can also fall back on the uses of humor (if he/she has it). Using humor is generally important in working with groups and specifically to building support. Professional education and socialization tends to stiffen our approach and seems to discourage both purposeful and spontaneous humor. Yet, appropriate and timely humor can effectively relieve group tensions, anxiety, embarrassment and facilitate dealing with pain and suffering. After undergoing heart surgery, for example, a blue collar worker was extremely concerned about being sexually impotent, but was unable to discuss this concern with his doctors. His hospital female social worker responded to the awkwardness by asking, "Are you worried about whether the lead has run out of the pencil?" Laughter, tears and a frank discussion followed.

NOTES

1. For discussion and illustration of the concept, see, A. Gitterman and L. Shulman, eds. *The Mutual Aid Group and The Life Cycle*. Itasca, Ill: Peacock Press, 1986; and W. Schwartz and S. Zalba eds. *The Practice of Group Work*. New York: Columbia University Press, 1971.

2. Acceptance is a core characteristic in C. Roger's description of the helping relationship, see C. Rogers, "The Characteristics of a Helping Relationship," *On Becoming a Person*. Boston: Houghton Mifflin, 1961.

3. For a discussion of the concept of support in social work practice, see, J. Nelsen, "Support: A Necessary Condition for Change," *Social Casework*: (Sept., 1980): 388-92.

4. For elaboration of the formulation, see, C. Germain and A. Gitterman, *The Life Model of Social Work Practice*. New York: Columbia University Press, 1980.

5. For discussion about the influence of group compositions, see, H. Betcher and F. Maple, "Elements and Issues in Group Composition," in P. Glasser, R. Sarri, and R. Vinter, eds. *Individual Change Through Small Groups* (New York: Free Press, 1974) pp. 186-208; A. Gitterman, "Developing a New Group Service: Strategies and Skills," in A. Gitterman and L. Shulman, eds. *Mutual Aid Groups and The Life Cycle* (Itasca, Ill: F.E. Peacock Publishers, Inc., 1986, pp. 53-74; H. Northern, *Social Work with Groups* (New York: Columbia University Press, 1969, pp. 86-143; W. Shalinsky, "Group Composition as an Element of Social Group Work Practice), *Social Service Review* (March 1964):42-49; R. Toseland and R. Rivas, *An Introduction to Group Work Practice* New York: Macmillan Company, 1984, pp. 124-29.

6. A. Gitterman and A. Schaeffer, "The White Worker and the Black Client." *Social Casework* (May 1972): 280-91.

7. For discussion about the concept of contracting, see, C. Garvin "Complementarily of Role Expectations: The Member-Worker Contract," *Social Work Practice 1969* (New York: Columbia University Press, 1969) pp. 127-45; A. Maluccio and W. Marlow, "The Case for the Contract," *Social Work* (January 1974): 28-36; B. Seabury, "The Contract: Uses, Abuses and Limitations," *Social Work* (January 1976): 16-21.

8. For a discussion of these phenomena, see, L. Shulman "Scapegoats, Group Workers and Preemptive Interventions," *Social Work* (April 1967): 37-43.

9. See, S. Henry, *Group Skills in Social Work: A Four Dimensional Approach*. Itasca, IL: F.E. Peacock, 1981; R. Middleman, *The Non-Verbal Method in Working with Groups*. New York: Association Press, 1968; R. Middleman, "The Use of Pro-

gram: Review and Update," *Social Work With Groups* 3(1980): 5-23; L. Shulman, "Program in Group Work: Another Look" in W. Scwartz and S. Zalba, eds. *The Practice of Group Work* (New York: Columbia University Press, 1971) pp. 221-40; R. Vinter, "Program Activities: An Analysis of Their Effects on Participant Behavior," in P. Glasser, R. Sarri, and R. Vinter, eds. *Individual Change Through Small Groups* (New York: The Free Press, 1974) pp. 233-43.

Learning
from Social Group Work Traditions

Margot Breton

SUMMARY. This paper raises issues that spring from the three fountainheads of social work with groups: the settlement movement, the recreation movement and the progressive education movement.

The first set of issues deals with the social self and the perception of individuals as members of social groups and cultures affected by the social, economic, and political conditions in which they live. The second set deals with the total self and the rights of individuals as human beings versus the needs of individuals as victims. The third set deals with the relation of the small group to the community and discusses the need to develop a non-narcissistic concept of mutual aid which would include both intra-group solidarity and inter- and extra-group solidarity. *[Article copies available for a fee from The Haworth Document Delivery Service: 1-800-HAWORTH. E-mail address: <docdelivery@haworthpress.com> Website: <http://www.HaworthPress.com> © 2005 by The Haworth Press, Inc. All rights reserved.]*

Margot Breton is on the faculty of Social Work, University of Toronto.

This is a revised version of a keynote address presented at the 11th Annual Symposium of The Association for the Advancement of Social Work with Groups, Montreal, October 26-29, 1989.

This article was originally published in *Social Work with Groups*, Vol. 13 (3) © 1990 by The Haworth Press, Inc.

[Haworth co-indexing entry note]: "Learning from Social Group Work Traditions." Breton, Margot. Co-published simultaneously in *Social Work with Groups* (The Haworth Press, Inc.) Vol. 28, No. 3/4, 2005, pp. 107-119; and: *A Quarter Century of Classics (1978-2004): Capturing the Theory, Practice, and Spirit of Social Work with Groups* (ed: Andrew Malekoff, and Roselle Kurland) The Haworth Press, Inc., 2005, pp. 107-119. Single or multiple copies of this article are available for a fee from The Haworth Document Delivery Service [1-800-HAWORTH, 9:00 a.m. - 5:00 p.m. (EST). E-mail address: docdelivery@ haworthpress.com].

Available online at http://www.haworthpress.com/web/SWG
© 2005 by The Haworth Press, Inc. All rights reserved.
doi:10.1300/J009v28n03_08

One of the most vigorous traditions in social group work is that of discussing and analyzing our traditions (Alissi, 1983; Garvin, 1984; Schwartz, 1986; Lee and Swenson, 1986). Calling attention to our traditions and what they imply for current group practice goes back at least as far as Trecker's (1955) edition of *Group Work: Foundations and Frontiers*, in the second part of which a number of group workers speculate on the future of group work and the need to meet the challenges of a rapidly changing world. Many points were made which are still relevant, but I signal only two. One is an admonition: "Now the task is to re-examine and clarify and deepen the effectiveness of our practice, relinquishing if necessary some of our familiar past, adding and incorporating the new learnings and the gains that have been made." The other is a warning: "The clarification of our own professional problems will progress soundly, only if we hold on to what has been the healthy core of our learning . . ., and see to it that it will be enriched. This enrichment cannot come only from the other specializations . . ." (Trecker, 1955, p. 377).

Both points involve looking at tradition not as the preservation of the past, but as the manifestation in the present, in whatever form, of prized ideas or behaviors–something more akin to the Greek concept of entelechy, a spirit that informs, than to the concepts of imitation or repetition. At the same time, we are reminded that we will end up having no distinct social group work modality if our innovations are inspired mainly from other "specializations" and not from our own "core of learning." In this paper I raise some issues that spring from the three fountainheads of social group work practice: the settlement movement, the recreation movement, and the progressive education movement.

THE SETTLEMENT MOVEMENT

The pioneers in the settlement movement chose to perceive people not only as individuals but as members of social groups and cultures affected by the social, economic and political conditions in which they lived. To this intellectual position, they added the moral one of calling for changes in conditions identified as unjust. They finally held the strategic position that the people affected by unjust conditions should themselves be involved in efforts to change these conditions, and they facilitated this involvement. One recognizes the three stages of seeing, judging, acting–a hallmark of modern youth movements as well as of present-day 'liberation' movements. Underlying the intellectual, moral and strategic positions of these workers was their genuine desire to break down the barriers that separated them from individuals who came from different classes or cultures, "making real friendships with the poor and learning at first hand their way of life" (Schwartz, 1986, p. 13). I raise two issues which relate to the awareness that people belong to various social groups and cultures, and to the desire to learn about people, and about social groups, and about cultures.

The desire to learn about others, about different groups and cultures is laudable but does not suffice. I think most social workers would agree that it is not good enough, for example, for men to learn about women; men need to learn from women. The consciousness-raising and women's liberation movements have awakened us to this reality. However, I am not sure how far we are willing to go in this type of thinking. Do we agree that a majority culture needs to learn not only about a minority culture but from a minority culture? That the powerful need to learn not only about but from the powerless? Do we agree that experts need to learn from lay people, and professionals from non-professionals? Do we believe that social workers need to learn not only about but from their clients, and not only about but from group members? We have to ask these questions, for it is only when we are willing to learn from the poor, the powerless. the inarticulate, as well as from the non-professionals and lay people and from minority groups, that there is in our work a real sharing of control, a real sharing of power, and a real sharing of agendas, to paraphrase Schwartz (1986, p. 24).

The reluctance to let go of some of our power as professionals may well be at the root of our present quasi-abandonment of work with social change groups. In their study of social group work practice in Montreal, Paquet-Deehy et al. (1985) found that work with social change groups accounted for a mere 7% of group practice, and they surmise that this may reflect both a "low priority on social reform in an era of budget cutbacks" and "an administrative choice to invest professional time in personal change groups, rather than in adult community groups." However, as their study establishes that in social change groups, the centrality and the control of the worker is much less than in therapeutic or individual change groups, I suggest that administrative decisions also reflect social workers' professional preferences for the exercise of more rather than less power. This is an issue I have discussed elsewhere (Breton, 1989), and it continues to call for serious attention.

Our attachment to the exercise of professional power may help us to understand social work's polarization between "people changing" and "system changing" (Alissi, 1983)–our humanist self-image longs for the latter, our professional ego demands the former. But understanding is one thing, breaking down the polarization is another. Guided by the spirit of the settlement workers' strategy of involving the people affected by unjust conditions in the struggles for social change, but informed by contemporary approaches, I propose we make consciousness-raising a feature of all social work practice. I do not mean that all groups, for example, should be structured as C.R. groups; I mean that conscientization principles should inform all our practice. Thus change would not be thought of solely in terms of individual change (whether in attitudes, thought processes or behaviours): equal consideration would be given to changes in the social, economic and political conditions which affect individuals as *members* of social groups, races, classes, cultures, and sexes. We can also, in the same spirit, learn from contemporary liberative pedagogy (Freire, 1973) to conceptualize our practice in terms of empowering, rather than of assisting or helping. Then we will see group members and encourage members to see each other as active subjects rather than as objects of help. This type of thinking is clearly part of the social group work tradition, but at a time when increasing numbers of social workers are once more being seduced by the "glamour" (Trecker, 1955, p. 399) of clinical practice, it should not be taken for granted.

As to the settlement movement's awareness that people belong to social groups and cultures, I assume that most social workers today are "systems-thinkers" and are fairly sophisticated in the knowledge of how larger systems impact individuals, families and small groups. But unlike the settlement workers of yesterday, we often fail to use this knowledge to direct our attention to larger systems per se and to engage ourselves at the political level, getting involved and getting groups involved in social and policy change efforts. We use systems knowledge to better understand, assess and work toward changes in individuals, families and small groups.

One explanation for this difference is that "we have learned to specialize by numbers" (Schwartz, 1971, p. 19), and that, our sophistication about systems notwithstanding, the majority of us still leave 'macro' issues to those who specialize in policy and planning, just as we leave community related issues to those who specialize in community work (there are notable exceptions, see, for example, Lewis, 1983). However, another perhaps more basic explanation is that early settlement workers took a moral position when they judged certain conditions as unjust, and backed up their moral indignation with action aimed at righting social injustice. We, on the other hand, have opted for a scientific approach to problems and have interpreted being scientific as being judgement-free, or morally neutral; like many other disciplines, we are reluctant to concede that any prevailing paradigm reflects moral biases (Kuhn, 1970). Consequently, though we are conscious of the evils of poverty, racism, sexual discrimination and cultural elitism, fighting these evils has relatively little place in our practice approaches. It is not surprising therefore that so much is written about individual or group therapy and so many social workers aspire to be therapists. The glamour of clinical work derives partly from the perception that psychotherapeutic models are more 'scientific' than psychosocial or social work models. But more to the point, I suspect we take clinical practice, and 'science' for that matter, as an excuse to play it safe and to stay away from activism and from politically engaged and politically committed types of practice.

The trend toward therapy should not surprise us but it should worry us. It should worry us that social work is becoming "a form of psychotherapy" (Garvin, 1984, p. 15) and that consequently the role groups can play in changing their environments has more or less been lost. It should worry us because in the final analysis, if our actions do not reflect our concerns for social justice, we are irrelevant to the poor, the oppressed, the minorities and the marginalized.

This analysis should not be construed as an anti-science statement. On the contrary, realizing that we have lost much of the tradition of activism of the settlement movement, we have to move on and find an innovative way of reconciling a scientific or objective approach with a committed, engaged and, let's face it, a moral approach which identifies and judges social evils, and attacks them in deeds, not only in words. This will require more active mediating roles in the environment, such as proposed by Parsons (1988, p. 43) who noted, in her analysis of a low income minority girls' group, that there is a "need for workers to learn more about how to reach the poorest children and how to mediate effectively for actual resources . . ." I believe that effective mediation in the environment ultimately requires that political involvement become part and parcel of our practice paradigms and strategies and that we will have to accept the confrontations at the professional, institutional and social levels which are bound to follow.

THE RECREATION MOVEMENT

As the settlement movement draws our attention to the social self, the recreation movement reminds us of the whole self. It reminds us that ev-

ery individual has the potential to develop and to be creative. It is a reminder that we neglect at great peril. This is a time when social workers
are faced with enormously complex problems and tasks. The world
seems increasingly populated by victims: children who are physically
and sexually abused, adolescents incarcerated in psychiatric institutions
by parents because of rebelliousness, throwaway youth who turn to
prostitution because they are hungry, women who get beaten up by their
husbands or partners, homeless families forced to live in abysmal conditions, men and women who need mental health services but are left to
wander the streets, old people who are forgotten by everyone, discarded
refugees with battered hopes, and many more. Confronted with this
misery, the idea that our work could have anything to do with the creative use of leisure-time activities and recreation may strike us as ludi-
crous; an idea that belongs to ancient history or at the very least to more
innocent times and places. However, when we forget that victims are
not only victims but above all are whole human beings with the same
potential and aspirations as anyone else for development and creativity
and with the same need to "find a fuller life in association with other
people" (Cohen, 1952, p. 198), then we further victimize them. It is easy
to become more interested in problems than in people, to find the victim
in the individual more interesting than the human being. And so we concentrate on the debilitating effects of victimization, and turn away from
a competency promoting and preventive type of social work with
groups.

We need to recapture our interest in "primary and secondary prevention" which, as Middleman (1978, p. 19) points out, earlier on distinguished group work from casework, and went hand in hand with our
"priority interest in the enhancement of normal growth." Recognizing
that growth stops only with death, this interest must apply to all group
work, not only to work with children–though I confess that I am troubled by our virtual abandonment of "normal" children and youth, or
more precisely, of the "normal" in all children and youth; I wonder if
unwittingly we are contributing to the societal negligence of this seg-
ment of the population, a negligence that is a sad characteristic of our
greedy age (on this point, see Kolodny and Garland, 1984; and Middleman and Goldberg, 1988).

Remains the question of finding a workable balance between paying attention to the victim (or the troubled, or the suffering, etc.) and
paying attention to the whole person. I am convinced that one of the
answers is to structure social work groups so that they are effectively
"democratic and creative" groups, as Grace Coyle put it. In a paper enti-

tled "Groupwork as a Method in Recreation," Coyle wrote that, "One of the principles upon which group work as a method rests is its conviction that one of the chief sources of positive fulfillment for individuals lies in the deep delight available in the mutual interactions of a democratic and creative group" (Coyle, 1947, reprinted in Trecker, 1953, p. 96). I want to emphasize that this does not preclude addressing the *needs* of the victim, but it forces us to consider also the *rights* of the whole person. Indeed to my mind, Coyle's language speaks directly to contemporary liberation struggles, including the struggle to be free of labels, for it declares that human beings have the right to fulfill their potential as whole persons, and that they have the right to experience the "deep delight" of participation in a democratic and creative group.

Therefore the way we structure groups is all-important, for a group can be structured so that the whole person in each member is invited to participate, or it can be structured so that only the troubled, or broken, or hurt part of the person is invited to participate. In the first instance, the possibility of experiencing fulfillment and "deep delight" exists, in the second it does not. We therefore need to think of innovative ways of engaging the whole person: these include putting aside antiquated notions of motivation (Breton, 1985); becoming familiar with a social learning model of growth and change (Goldstein, 1988); understanding, respecting and making use of cultural idiosyncracies, as well as accepting and dealing with the discontent, the resentment and at times the rage of members of oppressed racial minorities (Davis, ed., 1984). We also need to think of innovative ways of making groups milieus where people can "become," which means milieus where they can "do" (Middleman, 1983). This will involve relearning not to be timorous in the use of activities, nor to be afraid of having fun; it will involve trusting in the healing and growth enhancing power of play *per se* versus believing only in play therapy. This thinking may well demand a thorough examination of the assumptions which have come to guide much of social work with groups as we have turned to what I would call deadly serious forms of group practice. However, we should remember that social group work owes much of its vitality and uniqueness to the theories about normal growth and development and the attending orientation to the total person which came out of its early association with the recreation movement. As we face the challenges of a changing social context, we would do well to build on the particular traditions that go back to this movement.

THE PROGRESSIVE EDUCATION MOVEMENT

The progressive education movement was influenced by the emerging social sciences (social psychology and sociology in particular) and their early formulations about the nature of the small group (Cooley, 1909) and its potential for education (Dewey, 1922). It was also influenced by Dewey's philosophical positions on the ideal forms of government and his views on citizenship. Thus, the followers of this movement (among whom group workers were prominent) saw the small group as an experience that prepared the individual for democratic participation in the affairs of the community. The small group and its relation to the community is the focus of this last section. I deal with two issues: first, how we conceptualize the power of the small group, and what mutual aid means to us at the present time; and second, the relevance of democratic participation to group work practice in a culturally pluralistic world.

The sociological and philosophical interest in reciprocity between the individual and society and between the small group and society was incorporated into the first attempts at systematizing a social group work approach, when Grace Coyle (1946) called for a knowledge base that would include community relations as well as individual behaviour, group process, program content and activities, and supervision. The importance given to external relationships grew to be recognized as a hallmark of group work, so much so that Alissi (1982, p. 15) would write that unlike all other group methods "in social group work the group itself is taken as a natural part of a larger whole and is to be worked within that context wherever possible." Seeing the group as part of a larger whole (systemic view) is assumed to lead not only to a better understanding of the group, but to the group effecting the larger social structure (Abels and Abels, 1980).

Pursuing the concept of reciprocity, Schwartz (1961) in "The Social Worker in the Group" set forth his pathbreaking ideas on mutual aid. Since then the dynamics and techniques of mutual aid in the small group have been researched and documented (e.g., Shulman, 1984; Gitterman and Shulman, 1985) and application of Schwartz's ideas in a wide variety of settings and with widely different populations are reported increasingly in the group work literature (e.g., Lee, 1986; Parsons, 1988; Shields, 1986).

I assume that today any social worker who has taken even a single course on group work is at least aware of the group as a system of mutual aid (this was not always the case, and Shapiro (1977) called attention to our neglect of this phenomenon more than a decade ago). But I think it is fair to say that mutual aid is seen nowadays largely as an intra-group phenomenon; what is recognized is the power members have to influence and to help one another. I agree that the recognition of this power constitutes a *sine qua non* of effective use of groups. I fear, however, that reducing mutual aid to an intra-group phenomenon has led us to concentrate on the healing power of mutual aid and to forget its liberating power. Liberating power is linked to extra-group and to inter-group solidarity, which leads to strength, action and change at the social, economic and political levels. Intra-group solidarity, which is how we have come to see mutual aid, leads mainly to strength, action and change at the personal level. Concern with personal strength, action and change is part of the very fabric of our profession, but it is simply insufficient if our work is to have any relevance whatsoever to the poor, the racially, ethnically or sexually oppressed, to exploited children, youth and old people, and to all the others who are relegated to the margins of society, and await opportunities for empowerment.

Therefore, we need to challenge our present conceptualization of mutual aid so that it reflects all aspects of solidarity: intra-group as well as extra and inter-group solidarity. There is much in place already to guide us in this task, from broader theoretical building-blocks such as Germain and Gitterman's Life Model of Social Work Practice (1980) and the emerging Integrative Perspective proposed by Lee (1986) and others (Parsons et al., 1988), to historical and critical analyses of the concept of mutual aid per se (Lee and Swenson, 1986). We also can deduce from Lang's (1986) work on collectivities, Schopler and Galinsky's (1984) on open-ended groups, and that of many academics and practitioners on time-limited groups (see Alissi and Casper, eds., 1985), that the solidarity possible in these social systems, while different from the mutual aid which characterizes a fully developed, autonomous, stable and 'ongoing' group, can be harnessed for social and collective as well as for personal purposes. In addition, knowledge of network building as it relates to social group work (Abels and Abels, 1980; Shapiro, 1986) encourages us to think of solidarity between people as being more than a purely intra-group mutual aid process, and again to see in this kind of solidarity the potential for social as well as personal change.

Without these new ways of thinking, our perceptions and interpretations of mutual aid will grow increasingly narcissistic, and narcissism is dangerous in a culturally pluralistic world. This is one reason why our traditional commitment to democratic ideals and to democratic participation in and out of the group is of such importance at this point in time.

But we have to be ready to innovate also in this area, both at the conceptual and practice levels. We need to rethink "community" and ask ourselves what "community" means in a world where diverse civilizations, values and cultures collide in what have been called global cities and villages. We need to rethink "participation in community affairs," and what this means to the segments of the population that are effectively disenfranchised (Breton, 1987). To address these questions assumes that we are still interested in social peace and social justice, not only in peace of mind and mental health. To begin to answer the questions assumes that we are ready to drop narcissistic interpretations of mutual aid whereby we encourage group members to care for the others who are "in the same boat," but fail to awaken their consciousness of others in "other boats."

CONCLUSION

To survive, cope and find fulfillment in a culturally pluralistic and rapidly changing world requires an awareness that one's self-interest is linked to the welfare of the larger ecological system, not only to the welfare of one's immediate ecological niche. It requires a willingness to accommodate to philosophical, religious, economic, social and political views that are different from the views of one's own reference groups, without abandoning fundamental values regarding individual and collective rights and freedoms. This presents social group workers with a challenge which can be met providing we resolve certain issues.

I assumed throughout this paper that what makes social group work unique is its "combined focus on the individual and society" (Alissi, 1982, p. 10). Given that this assumption is widely held by social workers, it is an aberration that we have distanced ourselves from the social sciences (economics, sociology, social anthropology, social psychology), as well as from other disciplines such as education, forfeiting opportunities to influence knowledge as well as to be influenced by knowledge in those sectors, and have chosen instead not so much to dialogue with but mostly to listen to the psychiatric profession, and within that profession, to clinical not community psychiatry. I recognized earlier that action oriented toward social change leads to action at the political level and is much more risk-intensive for social workers and the institutions which employ them than action oriented toward personal change. Therefore it is to be expected that in conservative times such as the present one, the forces towards preserving the social status quo and thus towards focussing on therapeutic approaches will be greater than usual.

However, if we are to find innovative *social work* practice responses to the challenges facing us, I believe we have to introduce social change and political committment as an integral aspect of all our practice models. It seems to me that it is just not good enough to take comfort in the notion that *some* social workers *somewhere* are involved in community-sensitive and social action oriented practice, and therefore the majority can go on with forms of practice that are undifferentiated from individual or group psychotherapies. There is a concomitant and especially urgent need for research in social group work to focus attention on more than individual behavioral change and on more than small group processes that facilitate personal change.

We have in the social group work tradition a rich resource of wisdom and experience in working towards more fulfilling transactions between the individual, the small group and the larger community. We therefore have a critical role to play as a profession in making the new and increasingly complex world that is dawning upon us a better place for everyone.

REFERENCES

Abels, S.L. and Abets, P. "Social Group Works's Contextual Purposes." *Social Work with Groups*, 1980, 3(3), 25-37.

Alissi, A.A. "The Social Group Work Method: Towards a Reaffirmation of Essentials." *Social Work with Groups*, 1982, 5(3), 3-17.

Alissi, A.A. and Casper, M. (eds.) *Social Work with Groups*, 1985, 8(2).

Breton, M. "Reaching and Engaging People: Issues and Practice Principles." *Social Work with Groups*, 1985, 8(3), 7-21.

Breton, M. "Liberation Theology, Groupwork, and the Right of the Poor and Oppressed to Participate in the Life of the Community." Invitational Paper presented at the 9th Annual Symposium on Social Work with Groups, Boston, 1987. *Social Work with Groups*, 1989, 12(3), 5-18.

Cohen, N.E. "Group Work in Its Broader Implications," in D.F. Sullivan (ed.), *Readings in Group Work*, New York: Association Press, 1952.

Cooley, C.H. *Social Organization: A Study of the Larger Mind.* New York: Sehocken Books, 1962. First published in 1909, by Charles Scribner's Sons.

Coyle, G.L. "On Becoming Professional," in D.F. Sullivan (ed.), *Readings in Group Work*, New York: Associative Press, 1952. First published in 1946, in *Toward Professional Standards* New York: American Association of Group Workers.

Coyle, G.L. "Group Work as a Method in Recreation," in H.B. Trecker (ed.), *Group Work: Foundations and Frontiers*, New York: Whiteside, Inc. and William Morrow and Co., 1955. First published in *The Group*, April 1947.

Davis, L.E. (ed.) *Social Work with Groups*, 1984, 7(3).

Dewey, J. *Human Nature and Conduct.* New York: Random House, 1922.

Freire, P. *Pedagogy of the Oppressed,* New York: The Seabury Press, 1973.

Garvin, C.D. "The Changing Contexts of Social Group Work Practice: Challenge and Opportunity." *Social Work with Groups*, 1984, 7(1), 3-19.

Germain, C. and Gitterman, A. *The Life Model of Social Work Practice.* New York: Columbia University Press, 1980.

Gitterman, A. and Shulman, L. (eds.) *Mutual Aid Groups and the Life Cycle.* Itasca, Ill.: F.E. Peacock, Publishers, Inc., 1985.

Kolodny, R. and Garland, J. "Guest editorial," *Social Work with Groups*: Special issue, Group Work with Children and Youth, 1984.

Kuhn, T.S. *The Structure of Scientific Revolutions*, (2nd ed.). Chicago: University of Chicago Press, 1970.

Lang, N. "Social Work Practice in Small Social Forms: Identifying Collectivity," *Social Work with Groups*, 1986, 9(4), 7-32.

Lee, J.A.B. "Seeing It Whole: Social Work with Groups Within an Integrative Perspective," *Social Work with Groups*, 1986, 8(4), 39-50.

Lee, J.A.B. and Swenson, C.R. "The Concept of Mutual Aid," in A. Gitterman and L. Shulman (eds.), *Mutual Aid Groups and the Life Cycle*, Itasca, Ill.: F.E. Peacock Publishers, 1985.

Lewis, E. "Social Group Work in Community Life: Group Characteristics and Worker Role," *Social Work with Groups*, 1983, 6(2), 3-18.

Middleman, R. "Returning Group Process to Group Work," *Social Work with Groups*, 1978, 1(1), 15-26.

Middleman, R. (ed.) Guest Editorial, *Social Work with Groups*, 1983, 6(1), 3-7.

Middleman, R. and Goldberg, G. "Toward the Quality of Social Group Work Practice," in M. Leiderman, M. L. Birnbaum, and B. Dazzo (eds.) *Roots and New Frontiers in Social Group Work*, supplement #3 to *Social Work with Groups*, 1988, 233-246.

Paquet-Deehy, A., Hopmeyer, E., Home, A. and Kislowiez, L. "A Typology of Social Work Practice with Groups," *Social Work with Groups*, 1985, 8(1), 65-78.

Parsons, R. J., Hernandez, S.H. and Jorgensen, J.D. "Integrated Practice: A Framework for Problem Solving," *Social Work*, 1988, 33(5), 417-421.

Parsons, R. J. "Empowerment for Role Alternatives for Low Income Minority Girls: A Group Work Approach," *Social Work with Groups*, 1988, 11(4), 27-45.

Schopler, J.H. and Galinsky, M.J. "Meeting Practice Needs: Conceptualizing the Open-Ended Group," *Social Work with Groups*, 1984, 7(2), 3-21.

Schwartz, W. "The Social Worker in the Group," *The Social Welfare Forum*, 1961, New York: Columbia University Press, 1961, 146-177.

Schwartz, W. "The Group Work Tradition and Social Work Practice," *Social Work with Groups*, 1986, 8(4), 7-27.

Schwartz, W. "On the Use of Groups in Social Work Practice," in W. Schwartz and S. R. Zalba (eds.), *The Practice of Group Work*. New York: Columbia University Press, 1971, 3-24.

Shapiro, B.Z. "Mutual Help: A Neglected Theme," *Canadian Journal of Social Work Education*, Spring 1977, 3(1), 33-44.

Shapiro, B.Z. "The Weak-Tie Collectivity: A Network Perspective," *Social Work with Groups*, 1986, 9(4), 113-125.

Shields, S.A. "Busted and Branded: Group Work with Substance Abusing Adolescents in Schools," *Social Work with Groups*, 1986, 8(4), 61-81.

Shulman, L. *The Skills of Helping Individuals and Groups*, (2nd ed.) Itasca, Illinois: F.E. Peacock, Publishers, 1984.

Tracker, H.B. Group Work: *Foundations and Frontiers* (3rd ed.) New York: Whiteside, Inc. and W. Morrow and Co., 1955.

Group Work vs. Casework in a Group: Principles and Implications for Teaching and Practice

Roselle Kurland
Robert Salmon

SUMMARY. This paper examines the differences between group work and casework in a group. Examples of both are used to illustrate the distinction. Steps that are essential to maximize the value and benefits of the small group and to ensure that group work takes place are described and discussed. *[Article copies available for a fee from The Haworth Document Delivery Service: 1-800-HAWORTH. E-mail address: <docdelivery@haworthpress. com> Website: <http://www.HaworthPress.com> © 2005 by The Haworth Press, Inc. All rights reserved.]*

In 1978, the first issue of *Social Work with Groups* appeared. Receiving and reading Volume 1, Number 1, was exciting. Those of us who had lived for a while viewed it as an intellectual rebirth of a kind. Group

Roselle Kurland, PhD, is Associate Professor and Robert Salmon, DSW, is Professor at the Hunter College School of Social Work, 129 East 79 Street, New York, NY 10021.

Presented at the Thirteenth Annual Symposium on Social Work with Groups, Akron, OH, November 1991.

This article was originally published in *Social Work with Groups*, Vol. 15 (4) © 1992 by The Haworth Press, Inc.

[Haworth co-indexing entry note]: "Group Work vs. Casework in a Group: Principles and Implications for Teaching and Practice." Kurland, Roselle, and Robert Salmon. Co-published simultaneously in *Social Work with Groups* (The Haworth Press, Inc.) Vol. 28, No. 3/4, 2005, pp. 121-132; and: *A Quarter Century of Classics (1978-2004): Capturing the Theory, Practice, and Spirit of Social Work with Groups* (ed: Andrew Malekoff, and Roselle Kurland) The Haworth Press, Inc., 2005, pp. 121-132. Single or multiple copies of this article are available for a fee from The Haworth Document Delivery Service [1-800-HAWORTH, 9:00 a.m. - 5:00 p.m. (EST). E-mail address: docdelivery@haworthpress.com].

doi:10.1300/J009v28n03_09

Work had its own journal again, and this would help the method have another chance to be born again and take its rightful place on the social work stage. Some of the articles in that issue are as relevant today as the day they were printed. Margaret Hartford's article, "Groups in Human Services: Some Facts and Fancies," Ruth Middleman's "Returning Group Process to Group Work," and Emanuel Tropp's "Whatever Happened to Group Work?" each spoke of issues that remain important today.

Tropp had become concerned that schools of social work were eliminating or de-emphasizing the teaching of group work as a specialization at the exact time that there was a growth industry appearing and developing for groups. The statistics published yearly by the Council on Social Work Education for a ten-year period ending in 1976, were the realistic basis for this concern. Social group work was fading away as other disciplines and other professions were expanding the use of groups. Since a vacuum had evolved, it was to be expected that other forces would fill it. We would not be pleased with the results.

Both Hartford and Middleman discussed some of the results of movement in that direction. Hartford said:

> Another myth is that if a worker collects an aggregate, that is, gets people together in the same place and responds to them individually in the presence of each other, something significant and helpful will occur. It may and it may not. It may be good and it may be harmful for individuals in a gathering to observe a therapist responding to one and then another in sequence, but it is not working with the group and it is not maximizing the full potential of having the group begin to work for itself. It is, rather, doing what I call 'Aggregational therapy of individuals.' (Hartford, 1978, p. 23)

Ruth Middleman, in her article, discussed three issues that contributed to the lack of attention to a stance that maximized group process. In her view, at that time, one of the issues had to do with the continuing dominance of the helping person, and a therapy perspective that valued personality more than group theoretical constructs. The emphasis was on intrapsychic issues, and led to what she described as group casework, a hot seat pattern with the leader engaging in extended back and forth discussion with one group member while the others watched (Middleman, 1978, pp. 16, 22).

The "aggregational therapy of individuals" that Hartford described and the "group casework" or "hot seat pattern" identified by Middleman are characteristic of an approach to group work that we call "casework in a group." Such practice with groups minimizes the unique potential of the small group to help its members learn and benefit from the differences and diversity as well as the commonalities among them. Casework in a group is very different from group work. This paper will identify and examine the differences between the two. Examples of each approach will be used to illustrate the distinction. Steps that are essential to maximize the value and benefits of the small group and to ensure that group work takes place will be described and discussed.

GROUP WORK'S PRESENCE

As training in social group work methods and foundation knowledge about groups faded from the curriculum in graduate social work schools and therefore from the profession, caseworkers who may not have been trained in social group work methods at all often conducted groups. That they did so, and continue to do so, is in keeping with social work history. People trained in casework worked in groups with children and their parents as far back as the turn of the century, especially in hospital settings. This was even before the first group specialization was started by Wilbur Newstetter in 1923 at Western Reserve.

Historically, some of the foundation beliefs in casework and group work are similar, and have shaped the current practice. Newstetter wrote: "The underlying social philosophical assumption is that individualized growth and social ends are interwoven and interdependent; that individuals and their social environment are equally important" (1935, p. 297). The dual focus he described is basic to all current models of social group work practice (Roberts and Northen, 1976).

Prominent casework scholars also emphasize a dual focus. Gordon Hamilton, in 1940, said ". . . problems are both individual and social; a case is always a complex of inner and outer factors" (1940, p. 25). In 1990 Mary Woods wrote, "In our psychosocial approach, ecological systems and psychodynamic perspectives have become inseparable" (Woods and Hollis, 1990, p. 9). Similarly, Francis Turner accents the dual emphasis as one of the generally accepted, fundamental points which comprise a common core for all casework practice (Turner, 1974).

The generalized acceptance of a dual emphasis in work with clients may be one of the forces that gave impetus to the actions of the Council on Social Work Education, which from the 1960's on, moved "to find, elaborate and teach the generic and underlying pattern of regularity that presumably unified the direct practice method of social casework, social group work and community work. This effort was intended to define more sharply social work's identity as one profession" (Middleman and Wood, 1990, p. 6).

This effort, however, has been a disaster for group work. Since group workers always were a small minority of social work faculty, generic practice courses, by necessity, were taught largely by people whose expertise was in work with individuals and who had little or no social group work experience. The emphasis in such courses was on work with individuals. Birnbaum (1990) analyzes the results in his paper, "Group Work, the Spotted Owl: An Endangered Species in Social Work Education." In it, he describes the diminution of group work. To continue the analogy from the animal world, the situation was akin to putting a handful of guppies in a tank full of goldfish; the outcome was predictable.

Despite this, interest in groups has not died, and this is not surprising. "When viewed from a membership perspective, one observes that all social workers and clients, as human beings, are members of groups. Those groups may be large or small; they may be dyads, formed groups, families, neighborhoods or organizations. Membership is a fundamental condition of all human life wherever it takes place, and across all cultures" (Falck, 1989, p. 24). Even in today's times, the use of group process was listed as the third most frequently used intervention technique in the study of 142 mental health programs, and work with groups has emerged as a major modality for service delivery (Middleman, 1990, p. 1).

The problem, however, is that what is identified as social work with groups often is *not* that at all. Gertrude Stein's phrase "A rose is a rose is a rose. . . . resonates, and we know the rose when we see or hear the words. However, "a group is a group is a social work group" is not true and it is not necessarily the same.

Konopka, in her recent paper on work with the emotionally disabled, commented that in the last 25 years groups have abounded with emotionally upset people and are popular vehicles for treatment. But, she points out, now groups frequently are boring, suppressing, and run by people with a need for power. Group process has been used to enhance conformity. Dissenters may be humiliated. "Revealing" may be required, with punishment if refusal takes place. Konopka describes groups which are one-to-one treatment with the rest of the members acting as bystanders. She calls for a revival of group work with ". . . its basic grounding in a philosophy of respect for the individual, the skillful and gentle use of the positive aspects of group process and the goal of enhancement of the individual's power and capacity" (Konopka, 1990, p. 14).

One can take heart from Konopka's remarks, and try to bring them to being. A revival or renewal of this kind of group work is possible and may be occurring now. "Trends run in cycles . . . once again there is interest not only in specialized fields of practice, but also by methods. Schools of social work once more are offering courses in social group work" (Sundel, Glasser, Sarri, and Vinter, 1985). There has been a burgeoning of literature on social work with groups in the last few years. Politically, our efforts in expressing the need for greater collaboration, inclusion, and participation with both NASW and CSWE have been fruitful.

DIFFERENCES BETWEEN GROUP WORK AND CASEWORK IN A GROUP

There are major differences between group work and casework in a group. Some of the differences are obvious, others more subtle. The worker who views each member only as an individual and who applies individual personality theories and dynamics without appreciating or understanding the impact of such concepts as group size, roles, norms, communication patterns, member interaction and influence, and group stages, to name but a few, is obviously practicing casework in a group. Similarly obvious, the worker who allots time to each individual group member, in turn, to talk about progress on issues of concern, who allots time in round robin fashion and who does not maximize group interaction and mutual aid, practices case work in a group rather than group work. Group work requires the worker to engage in what Middleman and Wood have called "Thinking group (which) means considering the group as a whole first, individual participants second when initiating or responding to others" (Middleman and Wood, 1990, p. 97).

But sometimes group members can all be participating actively and group work can appear to be taking place when actually it is not. When, for instance, group members are actively engaged in aiding and offering advice to one member who has raised an issue or problem with which s/he is struggling, case work in a group can still be what is taking place. If, in such an instance, all the group members become "caseworkers" in an attempt to help solve the problem of one group member, then this remains casework in a group.

In a pre-vocational skills group in a day treatment program, Sara explains that she is nervous about going back to work. She tells the group that she's gained weight and that her clothes do not fit, that she's worried that she won't be able to get a job because of the bad economy, and that she doesn't know what to say about the gap in her employment history. 'What am I going to say I did for two years–that I was hospitalized and under psychiatric care and doing nothing,' she exclaims. On the other hand, she also says she'd like to have some money and that she feels useless staying home, especially when her sister pressures her to go to work.

Group members jump in to offer advice. Doris says maybe Sara is not ready to go back to work yet. Robert advises her to go on a diet. John tells her not to listen to her sister. Chris and Lisa suggest she 'go for it' and go on an interview. Frank tells her to lie on her application and say she was working in her sister's office. Sara rejects all these suggestions. 'I couldn't lie on my application. I just couldn't do that,' she says. 'And if I went on an interview and didn't get the job, I couldn't handle it. I'd be sick for weeks.' Finally, she says in frustration, 'I don't want to talk about this any more. Let's talk about something else.' The group then moves on to discuss difficulties Frank is having with his girlfriend.

Readiness to work, pressure from relatives, feelings of inadequacy, fear of failure, how to explain having been hospitalized–all the issues that Sara raises are applicable to other members of this group. Yet the focus is maintained solely on Sara. The group is active. In fact, six members explicitly offer advice. But the problems that are mentioned, even though they are highly relevant to all in the group and are ones with which many group members have had experience, seem not to touch the others as they try to help Sara. This is casework in a group, even with everyone participating actively.

What would make this group work is the "demand" that group members apply the issue or problem of one member to themselves and their experiences and situations. What distinguishes group work from casework in a group is an emphasis on the commonalities of problems and situations and the concomitant commonality of feelings to which they give rise. In group work, each issue that is raised, even when that issue at first glance seems to have no relevance to others in the group, does have applicability for all. The worker who practices real group work draws out that applicability and elicits the commonalities and asks members to examine personally the issues of others. Thus, s/he helps group members to view and to use the issues raised by one member as an opportunity for all.

A SEVEN-STEP PROGRESSION

To practice group work when one member brings up an individual issue in the group, the worker needs to maintain group work's traditional dual and simultaneous focus on the total group and on each individual group member (Newstetter, 1935). To turn an individual's issue into an opportunity for all in the group, a seven-step progression can be identified that draws on the problem-solving approach described by John Dewey (1910):

1. An individual member raises a problem/issue/situation with which s/he is concerned.
2. The problem is clearly identified by the individual and the group.
3. The problem is explored. As it is explored, additional information may be gathered from the individual about the situation. Group members need to really listen to what the individual is saying. They may ask questions about the problem and about the feelings of the individual. As they listen and question and come to understand the problem through the eyes of the individual who has raised it, they develop empathy and communicate that along with their understanding, concern, caring, and support.
4. The worker asks group members to recount situations they have experienced and dilemmas they have faced that are relevant to the problem that has been raised by the individual.
5. Possible "solutions" to the individual's problem are identified, drawing on the experiences of other group members that have been recounted in the group.
6. The worker and group members help the individual decide on a course of action or solution that s/he wants to try. The individual is helped by the group to plan how s/he will actually implement that solution.
7. The worker asks all in the group what they have taken out of the discussion that has transpired.

At future meetings, follow-up with the individual about the problem and how things are going is certainly a recommended eighth step in the progression.

If group work rather than casework in a group is to be practiced, particular attention needs to be paid to the timing of the third step in this progression, exploration of the individual's problem. Enough time must be spent in exploring the individual's problem to allow other group members to understand and develop empathy for the individual member and his/her situation. Only if they understand the problem that is being raised will they be able to recount relevant experiences and dilemmas of their own. Too much time spent in exploration with the individual, on the other hand, can contribute to his/her sense of being on a "hot seat" and of being "grilled" by the other group members.

In casework in a group, the third step in the progression is frequently rushed and the fourth step, recounting by group members of relevant experiences, is often omitted altogether, as group members rush to offer advice prematurely.

> Jim is a member of a group on coping skills in a day program for the mentally ill. Jim is a lonely and reclusive 29-year-old man who has trouble making friends. He has been diagnosed as paranoid schizophrenic. Jim lives in his own apartment. He frequently annoys the group by talking of masturbation and walking around with his pants unzipped, by making inane comments that interrupt the group, and by pretending to fall asleep and lying across three chairs during the meeting.
>
> At the group's tenth meeting, Jim asks a question of the worker. 'I want to know what you think, Debbie. Hypothetically speaking, suppose you had a friend and you don't have any other friends, but this friend every time he comes over he smokes pot or does a couple of lines of coke in your living room. I mean he is a good listener and is your only friend and you don't do drugs or anything, what would you do?'
>
> Before the worker could even respond, group members quickly jumped in to offer advice. Jerry immediately said he'd just tell the guy to get out of his house with the drugs. Allen said drugs are dangerous and this guy's no good. Pam said she wouldn't want anyone doing drugs in her house. Ron said that the guy must not be a very good friend. Will said a friend wouldn't take advantage of you or get you in trouble. Finally, Jim said defensively, 'You know, I don't really care if he does drugs in my house.' He seemed dissatisfied with the discussion that had taken place. Others in the group seemed frustrated as well. As the meeting ended, Pam asked Jim, 'Why did you waste our time if there is no problem?'

In this example, the group participated actively by offering advice to Jim. But obviously, the seven-step progression identified here was not followed. The problem was certainly neither identified clearly nor explored. The members' "solutions" were offered to Jim in a seemingly belligerent fashion without empathy or understanding. Their own experiences, relevant to Jim's situation, went untapped. The result was that Jim and the group emerged feeling highly dissatisfied.

The worker with this group felt equally dissatisfied and resolved to raise the issue again. When Jim did not show up at the next meeting she was forced to wait for two weeks.

> At this meeting, the worker asked the group if they remembered the meeting where Jim spoke of his friend who did drugs at his house. Everyone did remember it. She acknowledged that the discussion had been frustrating for everyone. The group agreed. She asked the group's permission to discuss the issue again in the hope that the group could be helpful to Jim and engage in a discussion that would be more satisfying for everyone. The group agreed.
>
> Jim recounted the situation. This time, though, the worker's questions and comments helped Jim be more specific. When she observed that this issue seemed important to him, Jim responded by telling the group, 'I don't have any other friends and having this one friend is very important to me. This guy I've known all my life. We went to high school together. This guy is a college graduate with a good job. He has his own apartment. This guy is somebody.'
>
> The group began to understand and empathize. The tone of their questions and comments changed from a belligerent to a supportive one. Jim's responses, in turn, became less defensive and more honest. He was now better able to hear the group. Even his physical posture changed as he sat upright and faced the group. Allen asked Jim if he was worried about the police. 'Yes, I am,' Jim responded. 'But I don't want to end the friendship. 1 don't want to get caught either with my friend doing drugs.' Pam asked Jim if he ever talked to his friend about being caught when he does drugs at this house. 'I told him it bothered me,' Jim said. 'He stopped for a while, but then he started doing it again.'
>
> The worker then asked the group if they could remember situations they'd experienced that were related to that with which Jim was struggling now. Ron told of a time a year ago when he told a friend who wanted him to use cocaine that he would not do it.

Others told of other situations–times they'd tried to convince friends or relatives to do something, times others tried to convince them to do something, friends they'd valued and lost, people who'd gotten them into trouble. All in the group listened attentively to one another until the time for the group was up.

At the next group meeting, the group returned to Jim's particular situation and helped him develop a plan to talk with his friend about his concerns. Drawing on their own experiences, some gave Jim suggestions of what he might say, of actual words he might use. The group even engaged in some role play, with Jim playing his friend and various members playing Jim.

STRENGTHS AND MUTUAL AID

Group work is a method of working with people that is affirming of their strengths and of their ability to contribute to others. In fact, the very act of forming a group is a statement that embodies the belief that people have strengths and can help one another. The process of mutual aid, unique to group work practice, takes place when members draw upon their own experiences and deep felt needs to help their fellow members. They, in turn, will relive and relearn through their own offers of help and they will be the stronger for it. Brown (1991) states this well: "For members to be able to share their ideas and feelings with others is a means of strengthening the giver *and* the receiver. The collaborative problem solving that goes on during this mutual aid can nurture group members, enhance decision making, and build more cohesiveness within the group."

Breton (1989) emphasizes the healing and liberating powers of mutual aid and points out that recognition of the process by which members influence and help one another provides a power that contributes a *sine qua non* of effective work with groups. It is such mutual aid, she states, that leads to strength and actions and change at the social, economic, and political levels.

The quality of the mutual aid process that occurs in a group is what differentiates group work from casework in a group. In fact, Middleman and Wood (1990) identify the worker's focus on helping members to become a system of mutual aid and his/her understanding, valuing, and respecting the group process as a powerful change dynamic as criteria essential to group work.

The worker's role is to set in motion a process of mutual aid in the group. To set such a process in motion is not easy. The possibility of mutual aid exists in groups, but that does not mean it will flower. Shulman (1979) notes, "Creating a mutual aid group is a difficult process with members having to overcome many of their stereotypes about people in general, groups, and helping. They will need all the help they can get from the group worker" (p. 173).

The worker who sets in motion the process of mutual aid takes into account the entire group as an entity rather than just one individual at a time. S/he appreciates that the group is composed of many separate and unique parts, each contributing to a whole that is multi-faceted (Brandler and Roman, 1991). S/he also appreciates that help does not come from the worker alone, but rather from the interaction with other group members as well as with the worker. "The group is a principal means for the problem-solving and goal achievement, *supplemented* (emphasis mine) by the social worker's direct influence on members" (Northen, 1976, p. 117).

William Schwartz, in his simple but profound definition of a group, specified the importance of the interdependence of the members to one another and developed this as a major dynamic for growth and change. A client group, he said, is "a collection of people who need each other in order to work on certain common tasks in an agency that is hospitable to those tasks" (Schwartz and Zalba, 1971, p. 7). The ability of group members to gain from each other, to consider, to understand, to appreciate, and to build on each other's experiences, situations, problems, dilemmas, points of view, strengths and weaknesses–these differentiate group work from casework in a group. Such ability, put into motion and enhanced by the worker, is the unique power of group work.

REFERENCES

Birnbaum, Martin. "Group Work, the Spotted Owl: An Endangered Species in Social Work Education." Paper delivered at the Twelfth Annual Symposium on Social Work with Groups, Miami, Florida, October 1990.

Brandler, Sondra and Roman, Camille P. *Group Work: Skills and Strategies for Effective Interventions.* Binghamton, NY: The Haworth Press, Inc., 1991.

Breton, Margot. "Learning From Social Group Work Traditions." *Proceedings. Eleventh Annual Symposium on Social Work with Groups.* Montreal, Canada, 1989.

Brown, Leonard N. *Groups For Growth and Change.* New York: Longman Publishing Group, 1991.

Dewey, John. *How We Think.* Boston: Heath, 1910.

Falck, Hans S. *Social Work: The Membership Perspective.* New York: Springer Publishing Company, 1988.

Hamilton, Gordon. *Theory and Practice of Social Case Work.* New York: Columbia University Press, 1940.

Hartford, Margaret. "Groups in Human Services: Some Facts and Fancies." *Social Work with Groups*, Vol. 1, No. 1, 1978.

Konopka, Gisela. "Past/Present Issues in Group Work with the Emotionally Disabled: Part II, Thirty-five Years of Group Work in Psychiatric Settings." *Social Work with Groups*, Vol, 13, No. 1, 1990.

Middleman, Ruth R. "Group work and the Heimlich Maneuver: Unchoking Social Work Education." Plenary address delivered at the Twelfth Annual Symposium on Social Work with Groups, Miami, Florida, October, 1990.

Middleman, Ruth R. "Returning Group Process to Group Work." *Social Work with Groups*, Vol. 1, No. 1, 1978.

Middleman, Ruth R. and Wood, Gale Goldberg. *Skills for Direct Practice in Social Work.* New York: Columbia University Press, 1990.

Newstetter, Wilbur I. "What Is Social Group Work?" *Proceedings of The National Conference of Social Work*, 1935, pp. 291-299.

Northen, Helen. "Psychosocial Practice in Small Groups." In Robert Roberts and Helen Northen, eds. *Theories of Social Work with Groups.* New York: Columbia University Press, 1976.

Roberts, Robert, and Northen, Helen, eds. *Theories of Social Work with Groups.* New York: Columbia University Press, 1976.

Schwartz, William and Zalba, Serapio. *The Practice of Group Work.* New York: Columbia University Press 1971.

Shulman, Lawrence. *The Skills of Helping Individuals and Groups.* Itasca, Ill.: Peacock, 1979.

Suadel, Martin, Glasser, Paul, Sarri, Rosemary, Vinter, Robert, eds. *Individual Change Through Small Groups.* 2nd edition. New York: The Free Press, 1985.

Tropp, Emanuel. "Whatever Happened to Group Work?" *Social Work with Groups*, Vol. 1, No. 1, 1978.

Turner, Francis I., ed. *Social Work Treatment: Interlocking Theoretieal Approaches.* New York: The Free Press, 1974.

Woods, Mary E. and Hollis, Florence. *Casework: A Psychosocial Therapy.* 4th Edition. New York: McGraw-Hill Publishing Company, 1990.

Group Work
with 'Mixed Membership' Groups:
Issues of Race and Gender

Allan Brown
Tara Mistry

SUMMARY. The small group is a social microcosm of the wider society in which it is located. Patterns of social oppression will be repeated in social group work practice unless active steps are taken to
counteract these tendencies and replace them with a culture of empowerment. This article examines some of the information available
about the effects of race and gender in small groups, and develops
some practice principles to inform a methodology for anti-oppressive
group work in 'mixed' groups. *[Article copies available for a fee from The
Haworth Document Delivery Service: 1-800-HAWORTH. E-mail address:
<docdelivery@haworthpress.com> Website: <http://www.HaworthPress.com>
© 2005 by The Haworth Press, Inc. All rights reserved.]*

This subject is beset with contentious definitional problems, and we
start therefore with an attempt to clarify our use of terminology in this

Allan Brown, BA, DSA, DASS (LSE), is Senior Lecturer and Tara Mistry, BA
(Hons), DASS, CQSW, is Lecturer in Social Work, School of Applied Social Studies,
University of Bristol, 8, Woodland Road, Bristol BS8 1TN, England.

This article was originally published in *Social Work with Groups*, Vol. 17 (3) © 1994
by The Haworth Press, Inc.

[Haworth co-indexing entry note]: "Group Work with 'Mixed Membership' Groups: Issues of Race
and Gender." Brown, Allan, and Tara Mistry. Co-published simultaneously in *Social Work with Groups*
The Haworth Press, Inc.) Vol. 28, No. 3/4, 2005, pp. 133-148; and: *A Quarter Century of Classics
(1978-2004): Capturing the Theory, Practice, and Spirit of Social Work with Groups* (ed: Andrew Malekoff,
and Roselle Kurland) The Haworth Press, Inc., 2005, pp. 133-148. Single or multiple copies of this article are
available for a fee from The Haworth Document Delivery Service [1-800-HAWORTH, 9:00 a.m. - 5:00 p.m.
(EST). E-mail address: docdelivery@haworthpress.com].

Available online at http://www.haworthpress.com/web/SWG
doi:10.1300/J009v28n03_10

paper. By 'mixed' we mean a group membership with a composition which includes black and white people and/or women and men. Our use of the term 'black' is that used quite commonly in the political context in Britain to refer to people from those ethnic groups whose skin color attracts a racist response in a predominantly white society. We are aware that in the USA 'black' refers to African-Americans and not to other ethnic groups, for example Hispanic or Indian. For clarity in the major argument we shall retain the inclusive term 'black,' but when the occasion requires it–for example when cultural difference rather than racism is the issue–we shall refer to specific ethnic groupings.

'Sex' and 'gender' tend to be used interchangeably in the group work literature (as in Garvin and Reed, 1983). We shall use sex to refer to the biologically determined differences between women and men, and gender to refer to the socially constructed meanings associated with female and male. By 'anti-oppressive' we mean practice which in Philipson's words '. . . works to a model of empowerment and liberation and re-quires a fundamental rethinking of values, institutions and relation-ships' (1992, p. 15). This paper concentrates on the in-group dimension of anti-oppressive practice. We are in full agreement with Breton's view that '. . . the times are such that social workers cannot afford the luxury of looking only at what goes on inside groups' (1991, p. 46), but think that in-group anti-oppressive practice is an essential starting point for social group workers.

There are of course unfortunately many other oppressions besides those associated with race and gender. We have selected these because of their centrality in our own experience and understanding, and be-cause we believe that many of the points made in this paper transfer di-rectly to other oppressions in the social microcosm of the group. Our view is that ranking oppressions in order of hierarchical importance is itself an oppressive act, and we recognize that each oppression merits analysis in its own right.

THEORETICAL AND IDEOLOGICAL BACKGROUND

There have been several theoretical, conceptual and ideological de-velopments in the last decade, in Britain and in North America, which form the background to the rationale for this paper.

1. The sex and 'race' of group workers and group members has a profound effect on group behavior and process. Although there is some disagreement on precisely what some of these effects are, there is overwhelming evidence from research to support the contention that there are major effects. Davis and Proctor (1989) combed the research literature exhaustively and produced substantial evidence of the salience of both race and gender in groups. Garvin, Reed and colleagues (1983), in a special issue of this journal on gender and group work, demonstrated the pervasiveness of gender influence on the differential experience of men and women in same-sex and mixed groups. In one of the few studies that examines the intersection of gender and race in leadership in groups, Brower et al. (1987) conclude '. . . the gender and ethnicity of the group worker (and all leaders) have an impact on group situations that may be of equal force to the variables we customarily seek to affect such as program, leadership technique, group composition, and so forth' (p. 147). In Britain, practice-based articles refer to the powerful influence of race and gender on group process and the feelings of the workers and the members (see Rhule, 1988 and Mistry, 1989, both articles by black women practitioners).

2. *Groups are a social microcosm of the wider society.* For some time we have thought of a small group as a social microcosm, on the basis that any small group will replicate the social-structural-political status and power relationships that are evident in the wider society (see Brown, 1992, p. 154). This view is based not only on research-based theory, but equally on our own separate and shared experiences as a black woman and white man in numerous 'mixed' groups. It was therefore with much interest that we recently read Shapiro's article *'The Social Work Group as Social Microcosm'* (1990) and noted his views on the implications for group practice.

In his paper Shapiro conceptualizes group members as entering a group, each with her or his own personal/social frame of reference. The effects of this are analyzed on the two dimensions 'Familiar/Stranger' (inclusion and intimacy) and 'Horizontal/Vertical' (status and power), with group members experiencing society as both their in-group and external environment. Shapiro envisages group formation as the intersection of these individual frames of reference, and goes on to say, 'Social group workers have a particular responsibility–and opportunity–to help members engage sensitively with both the content and context of their frames of reference and, through this engagement, to shape the structure and development of their own group as a "person/group/structure-sensitive" task' (p. 18).

We find Shapiro's conceptualization helpful, but it does not address explicitly the 'fit' between different member's socially determined frames of reference. For example, part of the black person's frame of reference is that they experience living each day in a racist society controlled by white people, and the white person's frame of reference takes for granted their superior status and power as a white person in relation to black people and all those from minority ethnic groups. Similarly, the social microcosm frame of reference of the woman group member is likely to be infused with her experience of male oppression, and that of her male counterpart in the group to be based on a gendered view of the roles and relative power of men and women in the wider society (but see later comments on the positions of black men and white women in relation to sexism in a white patriarchal society).

This 'fit' between socially determined frames of reference is fundamental to the evolution of both group content and process. The latter will reflect the external oppressive dynamic unless the worker's perspectives and interventions are specifically designed to develop and nurture an 'alternative' culture of empowerment.

3. There is widespread evidence of the efficacy of same-sex and same-race groups for women and black people, respectively. The group work literature is replete with accounts of the advantages of same-sex groups for women, at least when the group task is associated with issues of personal identity, social oppression and empowerment. In addition to the research-based work of Garvin and Reed (1983) and Davis and Proctor (1989), there are other recent publications (for example Home, 1991; Butler & Wintram, 1991) emphasizing the strengths of women-only groups. Home makes a very convincing argument that for women to experience groups which can combine both personal and political change, they need to be without men. She supports this by demonstrating how in community work groups men have often assumed leadership and control, and been dismissive of women's concerns, for example about child care and violence, as 'private matters.' The men have a 'macho' ethos emphasizing ends and not means, using 'male' language, and a group culture which is antithetical to the collective decision-making, power-sharing model generally preferred by women.

In *Feminist Groupwork*, Butler and Wintram (1991) have drawn extensively on their experiences of group work in two English Social Services Departments with socially/politically disadvantaged, isolated and oppressed women. They demonstrate how the groups focussed on women's understanding of themselves and their experiences, and how feminist groupwork can lead to potentially liberating interpretations with profound consequences for participants' lives and social actions. To have had any men in this type of group would have been both a contradiction and counter-productive.

Research (see Garvin & Reed, 1983) suggests that whereas women are frequently disadvantaged in mixed groups because their needs tend to get subordinated to those of the men (the social microcosm again), men often prefer and actively benefit from being in mixed groups. One reason for this differential experience is that the presence of women is 'used' by men, often unconsciously, to enable them to be more expressive and in touch with their feelings than they normally can be in groups of men. We say normally because there are now some men's groups which are specifically designed to facilitate men working at their own issues. Some of these are consciousness-raising and to facilitate expression of feeling and caring as an alternative to the competitive status-conscious ethos that typically prevails in all male groups (Sternbach, 1990; McLeod & Pemberton, 1987). Other men's groups focus directly on male violence and aggression (Canton et al., 1992).

Turning to race, the formal evidence (Davis and Proctor, 1989) is less extensive, but points in the same direction: that for many purposes an all-black or ethnic-specific group is both preferred by black members, and more productive, certainly when issues of racial identity, racism and culture are central to the task. Other sources of 'evidence' in Britain include: the campaign to create black sections in the Labor Party; the establishment of 'black only' organizations of social workers and probation officers; and support groups for black social work students on qualifying courses.

The views of white people about respective membership of all white and mixed race groups are not well documented, and probably vary in different contexts. Our experience in social work training is that white students tend to favor 'mixed' groups "to learn from each other," whereas black students accept mixed groups for general learning purposes but prefer their own groups when racism and white oppression are likely to be high on the agenda.

The message from this research and practice 'evidence' suggests that the grouping of choice, in many circumstances and for many purposes, for women is women-only groups, and for black people is black-only groups. Two points follow from this. First, in order to meet both gender *and* race criteria, we are talking about four types of preferred group composition for black people and women: homogeneous groups of white women, black women, black men and white men respectively. Within the black population as defined inclusively, the choice between black groups of mixed sex, black men's groups, black women's groups and gender-specific/ethnic specific groups (e.g., Chinese women or Jamaican men) will depend on group purpose, political perspectives and cultural traditions. Secondly, the positions of black men and white women, who are both at one level oppressor and oppressed, should not be thought of as symmetrical–as we explain below.

In practice there will be some situations where workers are in a position to influence 'mixed or not' decisions about how group services are offered, and they need to take into account the above points. There will also, however, be numerous situations where lack of resources, the context, and/or the task, result in groups of mixed composition, by race or sex or both.

Composition is often, and quite properly, not controlled either by group workers or group members (for example in small residential units, and groups whose membership is self-selecting from advertisement). Furthermore, to exclude someone from a group on grounds of their race or sex when no alternative is available because of a resources deficit, and/or when they themselves wish to be a member (and many women and black people prefer to be in mixed groups), can be both oppressive and discriminatory.

4. Social action groups and empowerment. In recent years there has been a resurgence of interest in social action group work on both sides of the Atlantic. As stated earlier, Breton (1990, 1991) has strongly asserted that it is no longer good enough for social group workers to concentrate on empowerment within the group, for example when working with disempowered disadvantaged women. She argues that internal process must be coupled with an external agenda of collective social action–for example in alliance with community groups–not only by group members but also by group workers.

In Britain, Mullender and Ward (1991), with other colleagues, have developed a model of 'Self-Directed Groupwork' which as the name suggests is predicated on group members being in charge of their own group agenda and process, with help from a group facilitator. The group task is to identify agendas external to the group in which the members have a common interest. Empowerment is developed as the group work method as well as being the underlying principle.

These social action approaches being developed by Breton, Mullender and Ward, and others, understandably tend to play down the importance of group process relative to the external goals of the group. However, as we think those authors would agree, attention to process is integral to successful goal achievement. It would indeed be ironic to have an oppression-ridden group seeking anti-oppressive external goals! Many social action groups will by definition have homogeneous membership and their process falls outside the terms of reference of this paper. Many other social action groups are, however, of mixed race and/or sex composition, requiring the careful attention to internal group process suggested here.

5. *The intersection of race and gender in groups.* A further complexity already anticipated is the interaction of race and gender issues in the same group. There is not much on this important subject in the group work literature, and we do not have space to make more than one or two points here.

One of the issues is the potential and actual conflict that can occur between these two oppressions. Many black women reacted critically to the white dominated feminist movement in the earlier days when it was demonstrably racist in its 'white assumption' and failure to address the racism which is central to the experience of all black women. The positions of black women and white men can in one respect be distinguished from those of black men and white women. For the former the oppressed/oppressor dimensions point in the same direction, whereas for the latter they are in opposing directions. Thus in a group composed entirely of white men and black women the dynamic is clearer than in a group with white women and black men. It is interesting to note that in the research of Brower et al. (1987) into (white) group member reactions to leaders of varying ethnicity and sex, there was more positive feedback about their experience of black women and white men leaders than either black men or white women leaders.

It would however be a mistake to treat the oppression position of black men and white women as symmetrical in Britain and North America. As Day (1991, p. 19) records, black women writers (Carby, 1982; hooks, 1982) have pointed out that the dominance of black men cannot be equated with the dominance of white men because only the latter is part of the patriarchical-capitalist inheritance. Day goes on to say that black women are not denying that black men are sexist, but that some black women identify their position as one where they 'struggle together with black men against racism, while we also struggle with black men, about sexism' (in Day, quoted from Carby 1982).

6. *Anti-oppressive group work is about feelings as well as ideology and theoretical formulations.* Inevitably much of the group work literature (with notable exceptions, see Rhule, 1988) on race and gender in groups is theoretical and objectified and does not begin to communicate the strength of personal feeling that for all of us surrounds the issues of race and gender. It is therefore very important when developing a mixed-group practice methodology to 'keep alive' these deep-rooted feelings in both workers and members (see, for example, Brummer &

Simmonds' reference to the hatred associated with racism, 1992)–
though not to the point where the group climate becomes disabling and
dysfunctional.

SUMMARY

There is extensive evidence that the structurally determined oppressions
of racism and sexism are replicated as a powerful dynamic in small
groups of 'mixed' membership. For this reason, among others, there
are many group purposes which, for women and black people and others from minority ethnic groups, are best served in homogeneous
'not-mixed' groups. There are also numerous groups, including some
social action groups, whose composition, whether by choice or circum-
stance, is mixed racially and/or by sex.

We shall now therefore consider some of the practice principles and
methodology which are essential if group work is to counteract the rep-
lication of social oppression in the small group, and facilitate the empowerment of all group members.

PRACTICE PRINCIPLES FOR ANTI-OPPRESSIVE GROUP WORK

The familiar 'good practice' group work principles go some way towards an anti-oppressive approach, but they mostly do not incorporate
the implications of the group as social microcosm. They underesti-
mate–or more likely ignore–the reality that, in a 'mixed' group, members enter the group unequal in power, structurally and interpersonally.
The homeostatic assumption of systems theory does not allow for these
structural inequalities. Anti-oppressive practice demands not only specific worker actions towards equalizing the power and position of group
members, but constant awareness and vigilance to ensure a consistent
approach to all aspects of the groupwork process. In what follows we
have necessarily been selective in our choice of which worker activities
to concentrate on to illustrate the approach.

Agency Context

While it is possible to work anti-oppressively with a group in an oppressive agency setting, this contradiction makes it both stressful and

problematic. Workers who are empowered themselves by an agency which is serious about equality and shared decision-making, are in a much better position to facilitate the empowerment of those with whom they work. For disadvantaged and disempowered potential group members, their perception of how the agency regards them will be a crucial factor in whether or not they seek to join a group (see Breton, 1991).

Group Composition and Structure

The general principles governing group composition for members have been well rehearsed elsewhere (Bertcher & Maple, 1977), and we have already discussed the importance of the initial decision on mixed/non-mixed membership. In mixed groups, a 'balanced' group membership (for example at least four black members in a group of ten) makes an enormous difference to the potential for an anti-oppressive dynamic. Conversely, the singleton member is prone to marginalization and stereotyping, and the worker needs to take action both inside and outside the group to create conditions which offer that member equal opportunity in the group.

Worker composition is an issue that attracts surprisingly little attention in the literature. The case for two workers is particularly strong in mixed groups (see Brown, 1992 chapter 3). As a general principle it is helpful to a minority group member to have at least one worker of similar sex and/or ethnicity. There is also the opportunity for the two workers to model an anti-oppressive, equal relationship between a man and a woman and/or between a black and white person. In 'Black/White Co-Working in Groups' (Mistry & Brown, 1991) these issues are examined in more detail, including the severe resource limitations on choice of workers.

The Preparation Stage

As in all group work, careful preparation is the essence of good anti-oppressive practice. Five aspects of preparation are particularly relevant:

- a location for the group which offers equal access to the group for all members;
- a group program which is at least in part negotiable, which in both content and methods does not replicate the dominant ethos of the

wider society; and which is reflective of all members' cultural perspectives and interests;
- ground rules which incorporate anti-oppressive principles about relationships and behavior in the group;
- worker(s) preparation;
- preparing responses to oppressive/discriminatory behavior.

The last two are now considered in more detail.

The personal preparation of workers (especially men and white people) undertaking group work with groups of mixed membership is essential. Theoretical understanding is necessary, but needs to be integrated with experiential learning which requires the worker to examine his/her own history and attitudes, and make a self-assessment of what he/she needs to do (for example for a white man to listen to what women and black people are saying about their experience, and for a black woman to learn how to cope with the feelings evoked by racism/sexism in the group).

With two co-workers, male/female and or black/white, the usual preparation for working together (see Hodge, 1985) takes on the additional dimension of acknowledging the significance of socially determined inequality in the relationship (Mistry & Brown, 1991). Especially in a new partnership, there is much work to do in honest sharing of feelings about working together, and discussing the implications of co-working with a mixed membership group. Sometimes a consultant's questions are needed to facilitate co-worker communication: for example, "what feelings and anxieties do you, a white/black person, have about working with a black/white colleague in a group in which racism may surface?" The pair need to work out together how they can organize themselves as a partnership in a way that neither perpetuates oppression nor overcompensates for it. Examples of the latter are when a male worker takes less than his equal share of responsibility in the group through fear of being seen as replicating the dominant male stereotype; or when a white co-worker is unable to query a black partner's actions for fear of being seen as racist.

The other preparation issue is anticipating how to respond in the group if and when sexism or racism–or indeed other oppressive behavior–occurs. It is clear that the worker(s) will have to be active and interventionist, particularly in the early stages, in affirming an anti-oppressive approach. Overt racist or sexist behavior is sometimes easier to deal with than the subtler forms of oppression, just because it is so obviously unacceptable–though often very painful. An example of one of the subtler forms of oppression is the gradual domination, often unconsciously, by men/white people of group interaction and decision-making, in the process marginalizing the contributions of women/black group members. With 'mixed' co-workers, the man/white person carries particular responsibility for challenging oppressive behavior, whether obvious or subtle, and not leaving it to the woman or black person to be the one who exposes the oppressive behavior. All these issues need discussion in the pair as part of preparation, with the expectation of revision according to what actually happens in the group.

Anti-Oppressive Work in the Group: Saying, Being, and Doing

From the moment the group first meets, the worker(s) needs to start establishing an empowering anti-oppressive climate based on trust. How they do this will vary to some extent according to the particular group model and purpose. Certain tangible steps on approach to program, ground rules, and the co-working relationship, have already been mentioned. However, though what the worker says is always important, the membership is likely to be influenced much more by how it is said, and even more by what they observe of the worker's non-verbal behavior–his or her being and doing.

For example, for a male worker to make 'impressive' anti-sexist ground rule statements in the group, and then to proceed to develop an alliance with the male members, tacitly rewarding their tendency to dominate the group, is simply to replicate the social microcosm effect of male dominance. Similarly, for a white worker to emphasize verbally to the group the need to be anti-racist, and then, quite possibly unconsciously, to undermine their black co-worker colleague's equal status role, is oppressive and disempowering of her colleague and of other black members of the group. It is a not uncommon experience in staff groups with just one black member, for that person to find him/herself marginalized by a cultural dynamic which makes it difficult to participate to his/her full potential. This can happen where there is a genuine staff group commitment to an anti-oppressive policy, and may be exacerbated by associated factors to do with gender, class and part-time/temporary employment status.

Research (Davis & Proctor, 1989) and personal experience both suggest that mixed groups–especially those with a gender *and* race mix–are likely to 'import' distrustful attitudes from women/black people towards men/white people, born out of a life-time's experience of oppression. This challenges the worker(s) to take steps early on in the group to demonstrate their commitment to race and gender being high on the agenda. Some of the most important steps are quite difficult to articulate because they are less obvious. They include: communicating non-verbally and empathically with individual members–particularly those in minority positions–through the kind of eye-contact that conveys recognition, awareness and feeling; being 'comfortable' in talking about, and the use of language about, race, gender, racism, sexism, and other oppressions; relating to a co-worker of different race or gender in a mutually respectful and equal way, without suggesting that anti-oppressive behavior is only a matter of good personal relationships; being prepared to challenge, and not defend, oppressive agency policies and attitudes; listening to and validating what group members are saying and expressing non-verbally; being quite open about recognizing power issues in the group, including professional power; being open and ready to acknowledge one's own oppressive or insensitive behavior when this occurs; acknowledging the reality of the social conditions prevailing in group members' localities, and so on.

Another anti-oppressive practice skill is recognizing and responding to the cultural diversity of members. This does not necessarily mean accepting, much less celebrating, some culture-based views (for example, religious beliefs that homosexual relations are 'abnormal'; the practice of genital mutilation). What it does mean is 'doing your homework' on the cultural perspectives of group members, and this includes class-based attitudes. Chau (1990) has made a major contribution to the literature on ethnicity, cultural difference and group work; and in the Hong Kong context, Pearson (1991), has drawn attention to some of the fundamental differences between Chinese culture and the ethnocentric cultural assumptions of much 'Western' group work practice-theory.

When workers have put their own anti-oppressive house in order, one of the most difficult tasks is knowing how to intervene when members are oppressive to one another in the group. The agreed ground rules provide a benchmark, but the worker(s) still has to make delicate judgements about when and how to intervene between members. As outlined elsewhere (Mistry & Brown, 1991) the tendency is for white and male workers, in respect of racism and sexism respectively, to prevaricate if not collude; whereas workers identified with the recipients of sexist/racist behavior feel the pain and anger personally.

In both situations the challenge to the worker is to intervene in a way which is strong and unequivocal, yet without provoking an angry defensive response which exacerbates the situation and disempowers both the perpetrator and the 'victim.' Part of the skill is learning how to expose oppressive behavior in a way which is not so confrontative that it creates a defensive reinforcing reaction. Wade and Macpherson (1992), who work with young male offenders in a day center in Inner London, describe the dilemma they faced in approaching anti-racism, in a mixed race group, with working-class whites who feel themselves to be powerless and worse off than their black counterparts. After discovering that direct early confrontation which did not recognize white men's feelings was destructive to all concerned, they developed a gradualist approach which included some separate sessions for black and white men on racism and prejudice, and which later in the mixed group enabled a more considered discussion in which anti-racist peer challenges began to occur. As in group work practice generally, one way forward is to make the issue 'group business' in the hope that working it through–painful as that may be–can be a source of learning and empowerment for all group members.

Links with the External Environment of the Group

In mixed groups, with primarily internal aims, an important practice issue is how to link in-group anti-oppressive practice with the external oppressive reality of many group members' lives. A particularly effective way in which this can be achieved is when the group as a whole has contact with the outside world as on group outings and in activity groups.

Mistry has described elsewhere (1991) an example of the power of shared experience on a group outing. The occasion was a three day residential visit of nine group members (black and white women offenders) and their six children to a holiday camp. Mistry was the only worker able to go. "One evening I attended a dance with other women in the group and we were set upon by white women holidaymakers. I was terrified, but the other black women (having always been on the receiving end of this type of behavior) dealt with it in the most skillful way possible. It demonstrated to the white women in our group how racism worked against the black women . . . and much of this shared experience formed an important focus for group discussion in the next twelve months in the group" (p. 152).

Another way in which the internal/external links may develop is when in discussion of racism and sexism in the group, examples are shared of the external oppressive reality of group members' lives. This in turn may generate external agendas for individuals, the group as a collective, and/or the workers and the agency.

Consultation

We are well aware that it is much easier to write about anti-oppressive group practice than to do it! Anti-oppressive work is personally demanding, and evokes strong feelings in workers, whether black or white, male or female, associated with personal identity, emotional pain and past experience of oppressing and being oppressed. The sheer complexity and strength of feeling can confuse perceptions and practice judgements, and sessions with a consultant can be a great help, particularly for inexperienced workers and for 'mixed' co-workers (see Brown, 1988).

In choosing a consultant, not only is their general suitability and competence important, but also their race and sex, depending on that of the group members and group workers, and the purpose of the group. As a general principle, in mixed groups a black and/or female consultant may be preferred, because they can provide both a support for black/female workers, and be more likely to recognize unconscious worker collusion with oppressive developments in the group.

A poignant example of the need for a same-race consultant is the account by Rhule (1988), a black woman group worker, of a group for white women bringing up black (mixed parentage) children. Rhule co-worked with a white woman colleague, and was the only black person in the group. The oppressive racism of the women in the group was such that although she had a racially aware and supportive white colleague she desperately needed to talk through what she was experiencing, on a one-to-one basis with a black consultant–quite separate from any consultancy for the workers as a pair. In Britain there are real practical problems of finding and paying for suitable consultants in these kinds of situations.

FURTHER WORK

This article has taken an overview of issues of race and gender in group work, and discussed some of the ingredients of anti-oppressive practice in 'mixed' groups. What we have not done is broaden the framework to include and discuss the particularities of other oppressions, such as disablism and heterosexism, nor have we done more than touch on the complexities of the intersection of race and gender in groups. These are subjects meriting further papers in their own right.

REFERENCES

Bertcher, H. & Maple, F. (1977) *Creating Groups* London: Sage Publications.

Breton, M. (1990) 'Learning from Social Group Work Traditions' *Social Work with Groups 13*(3).

Breton, M. (1991) 'Towards a Model of Social Groupwork Practice with Marginalised Populations' *Groupwork* 4(1).

Brower, A., Garvin, C., Hobson, J., Reed, B. & Reed, H. (1987) 'Exploring the Effects of Leader Gender and Race on Group Behavior' in J. Lassner et al. (eds, 1987) *Social Group Work: Competence and Values in Practice* New York: The Haworth Press, Inc.

Brown, A. (1988) 'Consultation for Group Workers: Models and Methods' *Social Work with Groups* 11(1/2).

Brown, A. (1992, 3rd edn) *Groupwork* Aldershot: Ashgate Publishing.

Brummer, N. & Simmonds, J. (1992) 'Race and Culture: the Management of Difference in the Learning Group' *Social Work Education* 11(1).

Butler, S. & Wintram, C. (1991) *Feminist Groupwork* London: Sage Publications.

Canton, R. et al. (1992) 'Handling Conflict: Groupwork With Violent Offenders' *Groupwork* 5(2).

Carby, H. (1982) 'White women listen! Black Feminism and the Boundaries of Sisterhood' in Centre for Contemporary Studies (eds) *The Empire Strikes Back: Race and Racism in 70s Britain* London: Hutchinson.

Chau, K. (1990) 'Social Work with Groups in Multicultural Contexts' *Groupwork* 3(1).

Davis, L. & Proctor, E. (1989) *Race, Gender and Class: Guidelines for individuals, Families and Groups* New Jersey: Prentice Hall.

Day, L. (1992) 'Women and Oppression: Race, Class and Gender' in M. Langan and L. Day (eds) *Women, Oppression and Social Work* London: Routledge.

Garvin, C. & Reed, B. (1983, eds) *Group Work with Women/Group Work with Men* special issue of *Social Work with Groups* 6(3/4).

Hodge, J. (1985) Planning for Co-Leadership Grapevine, 43, Fern Avenue, Newcastle-Upon-Tyne, NE2 2QU.

Home, A.M. (1991) 'Mobilizing Women's Strengths for Social Change: The Group Connection *Social Work with Groups* 14(3/4).

hooks, B. (1982) *Ain't I a Woman: Black Women and Feminism* London: Pluto Press.

McLeod, L.W. & Pemberton, B.K. (1987) 'Men Together in Group Therapy' in F. Abbott (ed, 1987) *New Men, New Minds* The Crossing Press.

Mistry, T. (1989) 'Establishing a Feminist Model of Groupwork in the Probation Service' *Groupwork* 2(2).

Mistry, T. & Brown, A. (1991) 'Black/White Co-Working in Groups' *Groupwork* 4(2).

Mullender, A. & Ward, D. (1991) *Self-Directed Groupwork: Users Take Action for Empowerment* London: Whiting and Birch.

Pearson, V. (1991) 'Western Theory, Eastern Practice: Social Group Work in Hong Kong' *Social Work with Groups* 14(2).

Philipson, J. (1992) *Practicing Equality: Women, Men and Social Work* London: CCETSW.

Rhule, C. (1988) 'A Group for White Women with Black Children' *Groupwork* 1(1).

Shapiro, B.Z. (1990) 'The Social Work Group as Social Microcosm: "Frames of Reference" Revisited' *Social Work with Groups* 13(2).

Sternbach, J. (1990) 'The Men's Seminar: An Educational and Support for Men' *Social Work with Groups* 13(2).

Wade, A. & Macpherson, M. (1992) 'Addressing Race Issues in Groupwork' *Probation Journal* Sept. 1992.

Waking the Heart Up:
A Writing Group's Story

Erica Schnekenburger

SUMMARY. The author examines the usefulness and therapeutic value of poetry groups with a chronically mentally ill population. A specific example of a group led by the author illustrates the beneficial properties of writing for people in a residential mental-health setting and the particular strengths and possibilities of such a population. Self-definition, self-expression, self-creation, and peer interaction are all promoted by poetry groups. The story further explores the importance and possibility of community linkage through artistic endeavors. *[Article copies available for a fee from The Haworth Document Delivery Service: 1-800-HAWORTH. E-mail address: <docdelivery@haworthpress.com> Website: <http://www.HaworthPress.com> © 2005 by The Haworth Press, Inc. All rights reserved.]*

INTRODUCTION

What follows is the story of a creative-writing group that the author formed and led in a residence for chronically mentally ill adults. The group met in weekly sessions of 45 minutes to one hour. Throughout the

Erica Schnekenburger, MSW, is a clinical social worker with Family and Children's Services of Central Maryland.

Address correspondence to: Erica Schnekenburger, 1413 Park Avenue, Baltimore, MD 21217.

This article was originally published in *Social Work with Groups*, Vol. 18 (4) © 1995 by The Haworth Press, Inc.

[Haworth co-indexing entry note]: "Waking the Heart Up: A Writing Group's Story." Schnekenburger, Erica. Co-published simultaneously in *Social Work with Groups* (The Haworth Press, Inc.) Vol. 28, No. 3/4, 2005, pp. 149-171; and: *A Quarter Century of Classics (1978-2004): Capturing the Theory, Practice, and Spirit of Social Work with Groups* (ed: Andrew Malekoff, and Roselle Kurland) The Haworth Press, Inc., 2005, pp. 149-171. Single or multiple copies of this article are available for a fee from The Haworth Document Delivery Service [1-800-HAWORTH, 9:00 a.m. - 5:00 p.m. (EST). E-mail address: docdelivery@haworthpress.com].

doi:10.1300/J009v28n03_11

seven months covered, twenty persons sampled this activity, with an av-erage weekly attendance of seven. The story illustrates, by tracing the group's life, the usefulness and value that collaborative poetry writing can hold in mental-health settings. Theoretical information and find-ings from the literature consulted are contained in footnotes where ap-propriate and relevant to the story. Specific poetry ideas and guidelines for their use follow the story. In the interest of privacy, some names have been changed.

I. THE MANOR

ARTHUR JACKSON
BORN 1921 MEMPHIS TENNESSEE
JAMES MONROE HIGH SCHOOL 1939
UNITED STATES MARINE CORPS 1939-1948
EPISCOPAL MINISTER GOD AND LAMB
KITCHEN WORK . . .

Arthur looked up from his paper. He was printing in large, dark capi-tal letters, forming a vertical list that covered most of the page. It was his first week living at the Manor; it was my first week there too. We were both "sitting in" on the Arts and Crafts group, at which over twenty peo-ple sat at a long rectangular table, coloring in identical photocopied line drawings of flowers, stringing beads, embroidering . . . silently.

"What is he *doing*?" one group leader said to the other. "His art is so weird. Ask him doesn't he want to color or something?"[1]

Arthur's list of the events of his life looked to me either like a re-sume–or an obituary. Alarmed, I began wondering what he must be feeling. Among 250 chronically mentally ill strangers who were now his house mates, who did not talk to him although they sat inches away; having been removed from his sister's house because she couldn't take care of him any longer; having lost control of the simplest areas of life such as what and when he eats, when he sleeps, when, where, and with whom he goes out, Arthur needed a way to say, "This is who I am. This is who I was. This is something I can control, that I and no one else can create. This my life, my story, my dignity. I used to do something. I used to believe in something. It was real. Maybe no one is listening anymore, but I still have a lot to say."[2]

I looked around the day room–this building did not look like a manor. The boxed four-story yellow edifice was transformed from a motel in the late 1970s as part of a nationwide deinstitutionalization which removed millions of mentally ill adults from interminable stays in psychiatric hospitals and placed them into the community. After the realization that forcibly discharging psychiatric inpatients with no provisions for mental-health services was unwise, large agencies such as mine set up "on-site rehabilitation" programs in these homes. A sort of psychiatric triage, our office was housed in a trailer parked in the service driveway and staffed by ten caseworkers.

The day room used to be the parking lot. It is enclosed now on two sides by floor-to-ceiling windows, overlooking a gorgeous park, and revealing today the kind of perfect sunny late-September day that beckons you to walk across Broadway and amble among the turning leaves and grazing horses. But instead, the day room was packed.

Residents sat next to one another in chairs that lined the walls, silent and looking straight ahead, as though protected by impenetrable shields. I thought, no one is talking, but, like Arthur, they all have something to say. Whether their silence signals sadness, anger, hatred, fear, overmedication, hopelessness, or language barrier, it seemed to me these needed to be expressed, and expressed freely, confidentially, with immunity, so that no one would place them in a psych ward, increase their dosage, tell them to "stop complaining," or even so much as say they're "weird."

It seemed to me that a writing group would provide many opportunities. By writing, people could create a letter, essay, poem, or story; have total control over what happens, and find a sense of competence and confidence. By practicing observation, description, expression, and communication, they could work to risk their viewpoint, better interact with one another, try to express feelings to family and friends, advocate to caseworkers, doctors, and administrators on their own behalf. By keeping a journal, they could problem-solve, and simply get things off their chest–privately. By joining a writing group, they could more easily make friends, find social support, and perhaps have a fun hour or so. Why couldn't such a group work? After all, we all have a story to tell.

This is their story.

II. THE CHILDREN

It's Friday morning, and all ten caseworkers enter the day room in a parade, with bags full of orange and black balloons and streamers. Without words, there is still recognition: If it's Friday and there are balloons, then it's the monthly birthday party.

The last Friday in October, though, isn't just any birthday party. It's the Halloween party, the day that the children from the elementary school up the street are scheduled to arrive in their costumes and sing Halloween songs. The day has been anticipated all year and has inspired such excitement. When are the children coming? Elaine asks. Should I dress up? Let me get some candy! Where will they stand? Residents lined up their chairs around the piano and sat there, not budging, even missing lunch so they'd have a better view of the children when they came at 2:00.

October 29 was a much anticipated day for me too: It was the day that I had chosen to hold my first session of the Writers' Workshop—at 1:00. I had spent three weeks planning and building interest in every one of the group's 45 minutes. And people wouldn't move from their seats.

"They look forward to these kids all year long," Sean, a caseworker, tells me over lunch. I smile. "I'm not kidding. It's a *big deal*. You think anyone else from the community ever visits them? They'd be happy if we weren't even there."

He was right. The community's attitude toward our folks was one of reluctant, watchful acceptance. "Outside" was for many residents a place where they felt, and were, unwelcome, eyed suspiciously. And so they stayed in, feeding this tacit agreement to keep themselves isolated and invisible. Yet the excitement and anticipation that built around the children's visit suggested the longing for things to be different—and the possibility as well.

"You want my advice?" Sean went on. "Cancel your group. No one will go anyway, I'm telling you. I've learned. I tried stuff at first too. After a while, there's just so much disappointment you can take. They won't even notice if you don't have it. Believe me. They won't go."

A challenge. I arrived back at the Manor in time to run to the loudspeaker and announce the first meeting of the Writers' Workshop at 1:00.

I walked across the crowded day room, my arms stacked full of black three-ring binders and boxes of ball-points. Thirty pairs of eyes followed me, curious. Six people—reluctant to lose their seats—finally agreed to join me around the table for the writing group. I—reluctant to lose my group—agreed that we would break as soon as the children arrived. Meet your clients where they are.

III. THE END

I passed around the notebooks, paper, and pens. "These are your journals," I said. "They are yours to keep. You'll bring them to group and write in them every Friday. This way you'll be able to keep what you write and look back on it over time. You can also use these journals as a place where you can say anything, anytime. If something makes you happy, or sad, or thoughtful, or inspired, if it was a lonely weekend. . . . You will always have these." No one touched them.

The group went around the table saying their name and an adjective to describe them beginning with the same letter.

"The End," said Elena, smiling in a toothy grin.

"Why does 'the end' describe you?"

"Because I used be able to do things. And now with my medication, I don't want to do anything, all I want to do is sleep. There's nothing left for me to do here anyway. It's all over . . . " She began to write in her notebook immediately.

Other members watched silently. "That sounds very hard," I finally offered softly, hoping others would empathize. Elena did not look up from her writing, as though a wall went up to protect her from finding herself sitting with a group, exposed. It seemed the notebook let her continue her emotional reflection, while giving her a safe place to share what she felt.[3]

"Wedded," said Walter, a long, gaunt white-haired man, his blue eyes beaming as he took his turn, smiling mischievously as he found his adjective.

"He's not married!" said Miriam, amused, sitting her small frame up straight. "I could have said 'married' instead of 'merry' like I did, because I am really married, or I was once. But not Walter."

"Hey, you never know," Walter replied, winking, again with that smile.

"Would you like to be married, Walter?" I asked.

"Was that a proposal?" said Walter, as we all shared the laugh.

* * *

It was an afternoon of surprises. Members spoke, were engaged; the laughter created a comfortable atmosphere. In the buzzing anticipation of the party, all members were asked to write an individual piece about Halloween, either present or past. At the end, members shared what they had written willingly with the group.

Most of them wrote journal paragraphs about waiting for the children to arrive in costume, about how they look forward to it. Elena, however, continued to express sadness about the loss of her vitality. After she read her paragraph to the group, members clapped for her, in a rare moment of relation. "That was beautiful," said Miriam.

"Thank you," said Elena, drained. "It felt good to get that off my chest."

"Sometimes it's easier to write things down than to say them out loud." And so the purpose of the group was defined and agreed upon by all, for now.

At the end, I asked members to put paper and pens in their notebooks and fill out their name labels before they left. Everyone double-checked in disbelief: "You mean we can *keep* these?" In a for-profit residence that controls the management of residents' fixed income, meting out an allowance of ten dollars a week and keeping the rest, such "indulgences" were rare. The pride and enjoyment with which they filled out their name stickers, decided how they would place them, where to put the pen . . . it was something to see. To me, well, they were just notebooks. But that afternoon, "just notebooks" became for their owners a symbol of respect, of being taken seriously, of belonging, identity, purpose.

Walter returned to his seat across the room to wait for the children. Sonia, sitting nearby, pointed to the notebook under his arm, curious but skeptical. "What's that for?"

"I'm in the writing group," he said, and smiled.

IV. MIRIAM

"I wrote two letters to my aunt this week!" Miriam told me as the group's second meeting began. She sat her tiny frame up eagerly with her notebook in front of her, practically shaking with excitement. "It was the first time I wrote a letter in ten years! My aunt was so thrilled! I told her I was in a writing class and that my teacher inspired me to write. It's all thanks to you, Erica."

I basked in Miriam's triumph. It was the kind of smile you live for, the kind that in one second affirms your whole existence. I suggested that we practice writing a letter to someone today, describing the fall day outside. Bringing their own perceptions and feelings to a common experience could help them not only share their insights with others but also become more attuned to their own perceptions, I thought. I asked Miriam if she would share what kinds of things she wrote about.

"Oh, things going on here in the Manor. You know, nice, cheery things. Not a lot of complaints. Just nice things. And then you think about the nice things, too."

Miriam certainly did seem upbeat and cheerful. Yet she'd had a difficult life. She was diagnosed as borderline in her twenties, and since then had lost her husband, her child, and her mother, and her career as a secretary, having been in and out of Bronx Psychiatric Center. Given to extremes, Miriam would go for a period of weeks to every group, participating actively. Then, in sudden overwhelming despair, she would recoil in anger and destroy any trace of involvement in the Manor. She would then spend time apologizing for her outbursts and be a "joiner" once again–staff had the cycle down by now. In my past six weeks at the Manor, I had seen so many things one might complain about, things that were not very nice. People should at least have the *chance* to say so, I thought–to get it off their chest somehow, somewhere. I told Miriam how I felt.

In a tone I hadn't heard from Miriam before, she began to yell: "My feelings are my personal feelings! No one wants to hear one long soap opera! No one! It's just not nice. So I'm not going to share that with anyone!"

I began to challenge her once more. Strongly, angrily, Miriam said, "No. I'll do whatever we do here in class, but my personal feelings are my personal feelings, and I'm not sharing them with these people. They're not for anyone but me."

Walter, Floretta, Lois, and Henry looked out the window, agitated. Not wanting any further disruption, I "okayed" Miriam until she was calmed, and nothing more was said about it. The group practiced describing the day, as I wrote their words down on a flip chart.

It was all nice.

* * *

Thanksgiving had me thinking a lot about my group, about what being away from family must have been like. I came to group the following week prepared to reach for feelings of loneliness and isolation that might have been amplified over the holiday.

"I'm not coming today, Erica," Miriam said to me quietly, the rest of the group seated and ready to begin. "I don't feel well."

"I'm sorry, Miriam. How aren't you feeling well?"

"I don't know, I just don't. I can't do it. I don't feel up to it."

Confusion. I had been practicing description with my group partially to help them express themselves more specifically than "I don't feel up to it."

"Even if you don't write anything, how about if you just come and be with us for an hour?"

"No! I tore up what I wrote here. I hate it here! I don't belong here! I should be with my mother! I can't do this! I can't take it! I don't know. Maybe next week. . . . "

Miriam walked away, still talking, and found a seat in the day room about ten feet away.

With the group's eyes upon me, agitated, I grew worried. I didn't want them to be "upset" any more. I eventually realized that Miriam was really saying, How can I trust you with all these feelings? Invasions of privacy were rampant in the Manor: There were no private rooms. Some staff would walk into residents' rooms at all hours without knocking, and they would sometimes search closets and drawers and scold residents as if they were children. It was so crowded–constantly so–that they would protect themselves the only way they could, by erecting defensive walls or not speaking at all. Trust was hard to come by. This issue was about the whole group, not just Miriam. Walter, Henry, Floretta, and Lois waited to see if we could talk honestly about this.

"So . . . how was Thanksgiving?" I asked.

It was nice.

V. FLORETTA AND MAMACITA

"Use words to paint a portrait of someone" was the exercise I chose for the group when it seemed that they were feeling comfortable with one another, less like strangers. As members called out words and I recorded them on the chart, it seemed we were arousing the interest of onlookers.

I turned to return to my seat only to find that it had been taken, while I wasn't looking, by a round, sweet, cherub-faced woman I knew only as Mamacita. During the three months I had been at the Manor, I had seen her only sitting silently, dozing on and off. She began taking my hand, saying, "Mamacita! . . . " every time she saw me. I took to doing the same. And this was all I had ever heard her say. She smiled and laughed as I cried, teasing, "You stole my seat!"

I passed her a notebook and pen, to which she just smiled, shook her head, and said "Noooo . . . " Though she spoke little English, she told us her name was Ramona.

While most group members decided to write about their families, Floretta, a no-nonsense 70-year-old African-American woman, decided to paint her portrait of Ramona. As the rest of the group wrote, Ramona sat silent and motionless, occasionally looking up from the notebook, smiling and shaking her head.

"C'mon, Ramona," Floretta said in her spirited southern accent. "*Write* something. You got *somethin'* goin' on in there! Just write whatever's on your mind. That's all *we* do. It feels good. It's fun. It gets your mind goin'. I talk more here than I do all week long. And you get a nice notebook. C'mon." Ramona's smile lit up as she heard the group's encouragement.

Floretta read from her portrait of Ramona at group's end: "She seems to me a person who is very nice." Ramona's first group, and she loved it.

Back at the trailer later that afternoon, I told Ramona's worker about the group. Ramona spoke no English, she told me, and couldn't read or write. Probably not the group for her. "Floretta can't read or write either. Actually, neither of them should be in the group. Talk to them about it."

But their finding the group—and each other—told me that they should. Regardless of their skills, they connected and helped each other. Their spoken contributions, which I transcribed and translated, were real, fresh, not overly crafted. They were doing it. And so I decided not to pass along the message.

VI. WALTER

Walter died on New Year's Eve. It was sudden. His brain had hemorrhaged; he was gone before the ambulance could even get there.

I told the group at the meeting the following day. Walter had died. I would miss his impish smile, the jokes he came to be known for, his laugh. Seeing him walking to the park with his notebook under his arm. I guess he wouldn't be getting married after all. My voice broke. Lois, Henry, Nobie, Miriam, and Ramona heard the news and were silent.

"I'm really going to miss him," I said.

Silence. Blank expressions.

"No one's saying anything . . . ," I tried.

Silence.

It seemed to me that for the people at the Manor, much was lost, much taken away. This was a loss I also felt very profoundly. I thought Walter's death could help my group begin to talk about not-so-nice things—to reminisce and remember and talk through the losses in their lives. And to begin to heal.

Silence.

"Maybe someone has a memory of Walter they'd like to share?"

"I don't like this, Erica. I can't stay. . . . " Miriam's voice broke, and she got up to leave in a hurry. I watched as the others got up to leave.

I'm hurting, not helping, I thought. My worst nightmare. I fought back tears as I headed back to the trailer alone.

VII. "HENRY, MY FRIEND"

"I like to write poems–about love," said Henry, a suave, 60-year-old Puerto Rican man who always dressed snazzily in slacks and sports coats. He was tall and thin, with a full head of brown curly hair and a brown mustache. He participated in no other groups. Instead, he liked to sit and smoke in his chair in the day room every day, smiling at the ladies. He refused to ever go outside.

Henry rarely read his writing out loud, but I always saw him end his love poems with a big heart with an arrow through it, rip them out of his binder, and fold them up tightly in his pocket.

No one else in our group had ever written poetry, including me. But the tough time we were going through led us to find another direction. We were a group, committed to one another. Yet we were caught in a cycle of my demanding they let me help them express these feelings; their being frustrated and resentful over having to, and everyone feeling frustrated as a result. We needed to create a different kind of atmosphere and a different kind of work. I read books by Kenneth Koch on teaching poetry and dealt with my initial fears. I decided to try introducing something into their physical space; to replace the blank page with something for them to focus on. This could elicit reactions using their senses; I would record those reactions. Henry was thrilled to begin writing poetry; he wanted to know why we didn't do it before February. He was the only one, though.

I plugged in a wave-sound machine and passed around rocks, seashells, and beach pictures. For our first poem, I explained, we would go to the beach.

"What is this?" Miriam looked nervous and unhappy. "I can't write poetry! I can't do it!" she screamed. "I mean, poetry is for people who went to college, and I never went to college. I did other things. I worked as a secretary. I wasn't–I didn't learn poetry! I have my Bible, that's all I need. I don't need this garbage! This is terrible! I'm not staying!" She stormed away.

"She'll be back," Henry offered, quiet and confident.

Miriam couldn't be persuaded to give it a try. The truth was, all of us, like Miriam, felt nervous, as though the very word poetry evoked all that was intimidating and incomprehensible to us. We had to be convinced that if we could feel, then we could write poetry. Henry persuaded us, "Try it. Just say what you're feeling. You hear waves crashing against the shore . . ."

Taking the cue, I wrote "Waves crashing against the shore" on the paper taped to the wall.

"Keep going. What are they like? How do they make you feel?" I said.

"Tremendous waves," said Lorraine, who was sitting by the wall near the table. "They bring themselves to the shore, one, after the other, after the other. . . . Oh, I hope you don't mind my joining in. I grew up by the beach on Long Island, and so this is bringing back a lot of memories."

"Right?" said Lois. "It does for me, too, of the seashells in the sand. . . ."

"Close your eyes," I said, writing feverishly. "What are you doing?"

"I pick them up and hold them to my ear . . . "

We continued, eliciting such strong and immediate reactions which easily led to the expression of memories and feelings. When we decided to end, I read the lines I had taken down on the paper taped to the wall. Memories were evoked:

> I pick the shells up and hold them to my ear
> and I can hear the ocean.

Senses were activated:

> Cool breeze coming from the ocean
> Open my shirt and feel the sunshine.

Feelings unfolded:

> Looking out onto the horizon,
> I want to go on an adventure.

And they understood themselves better by sharing genuine, honest reactions.[4] As I finished reading, the group erupted in spontaneous applause. We could not believe what we had built together. We had done something we never thought we could do.

"This has brought me back to my childhood, growing up on the beach," Lorraine said. "I did all those things–collected seashells, listened to the waves, took long walks. I haven't done that in a long time. I miss those days. This afternoon, I won't be hearing the noise here in the Manor . . . I'll be hearing the sound of the waves.[5] Those days are gone. It's sad. I've never told this to anyone here."[6]

The following weeks, I thought more creatively about activating the senses; I collected ideas from Kenneth Koch[7] and other poets. One March day I brought in a big bouquet of flowers and set it in the center of the table. Seeing this, Miriam joined us once again to try it. She ended up contributing the lines,

> How I love the smell,
> the beautiful red color
> raging up my senses.

Lois followed,

> The roses are out now,
> Bringing love
> Spring must be in the air.

Miriam, as though understanding her own struggles and the group's life, said, "The seasons come, and the seasons go, and there's always spring to look forward to." I looked over and saw Ramona beginning to write and draw in her notebook.

One week I brought in classical music and flooded the Manor with it, inspiring Sonia to come over from across the day room and begin dancing near our table. As a young woman, she told us, she had danced in *Carousel* on Broadway. She contributed the lines,

> It's the music that makes me dance
> I am entranced and elated.

Thrilled, I quickly grabbed my camera. "Oh, get away from me with that thing!" Sonia said, disgusted. "What are you doing? I look terrible. You don't wear makeup or your nice clothes *here. Ecchh*. I don't want a picture of me here." Looking back at the group, I saw only five sets of hands: Members went flying under the table after seeing the camera. Sonia sat down with the group after they shared the laugh. That day, the music brought back stories of learning to dance and courting that members wanted to tell one another. Back when they did want their picture taken.

One week I dragged over the solid colored balls from the billiard table; I asked for images and feelings that certain colors evoked. Henry offered,

> My favorite color is navy blue
> like a good-quality suit with stripes
> and I don't mean polyester
> but silk, with a silk shirt and a silk tie.

The group roared with laughter and applause at this, realizing that the essence of Henry had finally–definitively–been captured and expressed to us.

A photograph of a waterfall inspired Henry and Miriam to collaborate on the lines,

> A waterfall
> Comes from high up and falls down
> In a million love stories.

Members were surprised, at first, to see their utterances being recorded on the large sheet of paper, to see their viewpoints accepted, worthwhile, "right."

"Oh, you're going to write *that* down?" was something I heard an awful lot.

"Yes–just wait until it's done. If you want, you can take it out then," I'd say. They never did.

As the weeks went by, members spoke more confidently and freely. They began to trust in their own feelings and reactions; they began to trust in other members to be able to hear and accept them. The poem that asked them to describe what they do in the writing group contained the lines:

> Give my opinion
> Smell the roses
> Just by writing about it
> You feel the feeling
> and see the beauty

Conflict arose. Miriam took issue with Henry when he said that flowers were "like babies in the womb, soft and silky." The two of them argued the point, its meaning, and argued to me about its place in the group poem. They were ready to assume a greater responsibility for the group. It was a sign of growth that they could challenge each other respectfully, rather than withdraw and walk away in anger.[8] They knew they, and the group, would survive the conflict. This was possible because they felt respected. They were respected. Finally, they reached a compromise: Miriam agreed to keep the line in the group's poem if she could copy the poem in her journal without it. She discovered her own response through the exploration of others; she got to know herself better, and so could open herself to others.[9] At the session's end, I suggested members give their flowers to someone special to them. Miriam gave hers to Henry, saying, "This is for you, Henry, my friend."

Members grew to trust the group and the process, knowing that each week by 2:00 we would have written a poem–and done it together. The group gained respect and admiration: Over time other residents were attracted by the activity, by watching the lively responses and the poem taking form right there on the wall. They frequently joined in, as Lorraine did on hearing the ocean.

One week, we wrote a poem about the writing group: "Paint a picture of the group. What are we doing?" Ramona, who was once so silent and sleepy, gave the first line in her raspy voice:
"Waking the heart up."
Henry contributed:

> By putting the word on paper
> it is beautiful, like a rose.

And as I reflected on my work with this group, I thought, people are also like roses. Some open up quickly, some slowly, some never at all. They cannot be opened by another. All I can do is help cultivate and create an atmosphere that will make it safe to happen. And when it does, respect, appreciate, and admire.

VIII. OVER THERE

"I can't make it over there to meet with you this week," my supervisor had told me, referring to the Manor. So that April afternoon I waited outside her office in the administrative building across town. Some clients came to this building to attend day programs. Although I worked for this agency, I barely knew this building or these programs. The clients in on-site rehab, my clients, were considered the lowest functioning, unable to commit to outside programs. It was easy to feel disconnected and for-gotten "over there."

Waiting, I saw a notice on the bulletin board: "Perspectives in Recov-ery": The Second Annual Statewide Art Show for Mental Health, a cel-ebration of the talents and abilities of people with mental illness. "We are calling for submissions of painting, drawing, photography, and po-etry by mental-health consumers in New York. All submissions will be on exhibit at the Legislative Office Building in Albany May 23 to 27; all will compete for a prize. All poems must be typed and framed. Deadline for submission: April 28." One week away.

Joyce, the regional director, walked in. "How long has this been here?" I asked her, pointing to the notice.

"I don't know–a few weeks, I guess," she said.

"We never got it at the Manor–did it get lost?"

"No," she answered. "We just didn't think you'd have anything over there."

IX. ALBANY

I got back to the Manor and called an emergency meeting of the Writ-ers' Workshop. In an excited discussion we decided upon which poems to submit and planned how to present them. Sonia suggested that "A Myriad of Colors" be typed with each paragraph printed in the color it represented. We talked about attending the exhibit. Henry, who never left the Manor, expressed concern about such a long trip.

"Henry, you must come with us," said Nobie. "Please. We'll buy you a new suit."

* * *

"*No one's* ready?" Larry, the van driver, said in exasperated disbelief as he entered the day room on the sunny morning of May 24. The Big Day. We were supposed to be on the road by now.

Henry couldn't make it. He said he did not know anything about this trip to Albany, he was not told about it, and he could not make it today. He had to stay in the Manor.

We reminded Henry of all we had been through together. It was Henry, after all, who brought us poetry in the first place. We were doing work we never thought we could do. And now we were going to see our poems on display in the capital of New York. People from all over would admire our work, would admire us. Let's go show everyone what we can do.

"I have to go upstairs," Henry said, and disappeared. We discussed who should go up and talk to him some more. A few moments later he reappeared–in his brown suit.

"Let's go."

* * *

Lois, Nobie, Sonia, and Henry stood in awe of the grandness of the exhibit in the Legislative Building. "I didn't know the world was so big," Henry said. Thirty-three counties were represented in over six hundred works of art, photography, and poetry.

"I think I see ours!" I said, my heart pounding. The group rushed over to find our poem "A Myriad of Colors," a big pink ribbon hanging from it: "Honorable Mention." One of five awards for over sixty poems.

"Hey! Get our picture in front of it!" yelled Sonia. This day, no one flew under the table.

THE POEMS OF THE WRITERS' WORKSHOP

The following is a sampling of the collaborative poetry the group completed, with guidelines for practical implementation that is responsive to the needs, and strengths, of clients with mental illness. By including these examples the author seeks to inspire, support, and encourage those who might consider incorporating creative activities in their practice.

Poems Written While Looking at Photographs

I Remember Humacao
A rocking chair
How I love a rocking chair
Like the one my parents had in Puerto Rico
The view is terrific
In the country, life is peaceful
Six o'clock in the morning on the porch
A woman puts her feet up on the table and is reading
Tells me I should get out more

and not stay inside so much
Time is endless.

Photographs provided an excellent engagement tool with which to begin writing poetry. I brought in pictures that I had taken and enlarged; the size helped the group focus their attention on the details of what was taking place. Reactions came through immediately and were genuine and real. I asked members to describe in detail the scene, colors, actions taking place. Picture yourselves being there. What does it feel like? Smell like? Sound like? Taste like? Does the scene remind you of anything? What are you doing?

Members engaged in negotiating the scene taking place, and there was frequently disagreement. It was crucial that I not "solve the problem" by telling them exactly what was happening when I took the photograph. The group's task was to puzzle out the scene and risk offering their own viewpoints, learning that difference is acceptable. The impressionistic structure of the poems therefore reflects a scene as it unfolds, as it is taken in and understood. The activation of memories encouraged members to share certain life experiences with the group and led them to discover the commonalities among them. As one member allowed himself to picture the ideal, he began to problem-solve regarding the here-and-now of his own life ("Tells me I should get outside more, and not stay inside so much . . . "). Members can bring in pictures that inspire them as well.

Being Something Else (Written While Looking at Photographs)

I fly
East, west, north, south
Finding things to eat
I am flying faster and faster through the air
It's better than walking, isn't it?

I am growing
My leaves come out
The sun and the water open me up
Summertime makes me stronger
I feel lovely
I feel beautiful
I feel better than before

Members looked at photographs–first of a seagull and then of a tulip–and were asked to become those things. Write using the first-person, I said, describing the scene from your point of view. At first the group may have difficulty using "I" rather than "it." If the worker helps lead the visualization, members may begin to feel liberated, validate their unique perceptions, and tap into their sense of adventure and playfulness. Feelings attributed to others often convey the most wistful imaginings of clients who have been inactive and restricted. Having to express feelings from another's point of view can help provide clients with a nonthreatening vehicle for tuning in to their own emotions and perceptions, and for finding words to relate them to the world.

Sound

> Waves hitting the shore
> Tremendous waves bring themselves to the shore
> One, after the other, after the other. . . .
> Seashells in the sand
> I pick them up and hold them to my ear
> and I can hear the ocean.
> I swim,
> I find a skipping stone and throw it in the water
> It skims over the top.
> Waves are crashing against the rocks.
> The sunset,
> yellow and orange and red
> The clouds,
> bluish gray
> Looking out onto the horizon,
> I want to go on an adventure.
> Waves come in loud and brisk
> and wash out so softly
> leaving shells for me to save
> Rocks sparkle in the sun
> The seagull likes to look at the waves
> and the fish and oysters and starfish
> Cool breeze coming from the ocean
> Open my shirt and feel the sunshine.

I set up a wave-sound machine, turned on a fan, and brought in rocks, sand, shells, and beach photographs–total immersion. I asked, What do you hear? What do you see? Any colors, scenes? What do you feel? What are you doing? Members used the props to make the scene real for them, to evoke childhood memories, and to express their longing for a world as limitless as the horizon. Homebound people might be able to share the pain of their isolation; they may be inspired to go outside again. The sound of the waves also aroused the curiosity and participation of new members. Any of the recordings available now that capture the sounds of nature are effective in helping make an imaginary experience real for those who think concretely.

A Myriad of Colors
Green leaves, green grass
The beginning of springtime
dark and vibrant

Red roses, red dress
seductive and happy
The hot color of the early-morning sky

Orange is a tangerine
Beautiful and pure
Sweet and delectable

My favorite color is navy blue
Like a good-quality suit with stripes
And I don't mean polyester
but silk, with a silk shirt and a silk tie

The blue sky, blue eyes
Melt into your soul
I don't know, there's just something about blue eyes
My blue Yankees cap–it wears nice
I put it on and I feel allright

Purple cueball on the pool table
The color of the King's robe
majestic, with dignity
Pansy flowers, a delicate purple
A tasty purple grape

Gray, like clouds when the rain is about to come down
Makes me feel lost and disconsolate.

Colors give life to all creation.

I took solid colored billiard balls and passed them one by one around the table. I asked the group to throw out the images and emotions that the color brings to mind. I called for the most vivid adjectives they could think of and specific, unusual examples. This is challenging, so it might work best with a group that has already been writing poetry. The repetitive cycle of writing until the ball had gone around once helped create a pleasing sense of rhythm, adding to its dreamlike quality.

Experience Poems

Poems that evaluate the experience of an individual or a group are valuable for many different purposes and a variety of situations. As our group began to plan the synthesis of a book of our poems, I suggested we write a poem "painting a picture" of ourselves to present to readers who we are and what we do–effectively, to tell our story. They wrote:

Waking the heart up
Feeling better
Like whistling
Pick a topic
Enlarge on it
Describe it
Build around it
Work around it
Give my opinion
Smell the roses
Just by writing about it
You feel the feeling
and see the beauty
By putting the word on paper
It is beautiful, like a rose

Because this activity took place toward the end of our group's life, members used the poem to evaluate the experience, realize and express growth, and reminisce on memorable past sessions. Such reflection is wonderful if they had initially doubted they could write poetry. Too often, past orientation highlights only what has been lost. Helping members articulate areas of growth allows the group to celebrate together the gains that were made–together. Integrating the group experience also helps clients who have had painful separations and may have difficulty accepting termination.

The evaluative poem can also be useful in beginnings and middles. Members can collaborate to form a common understanding of the group's purpose, content, and goals. Feedback can be given and received; expectations for the future can come out. There is social pressure not to express criticism in mental-health settings, and internal psychic pressure not to expect anything at all.

NOTES

1. Where opportunities for creative activities do exist in mental-health settings, they are often used unpurposefully. Mann et al. (1993) establish that staff on inpatient units and in residences are often unsure how to provide therapeutic, nonstressful, structured activity schedules for schizophrenic inpatients.

2. Robert Coles portrays his experience in working with schizophrenics in *A Call for Stories*. He establishes that reaching for the stories in clients helps practitioners bridge the gap between them.

3. Artistic pursuits are inherently therapeutic, Rudolf Arhneim writes, offering "in the physical world a safe replacement of the threatening social reality." See his article "The Artistry of Psychotics" in *American Scientist* Vol. 74 for more on the use of creative activities with a psychiatric population.

4. One key benefit of poetry writing for those with mental illness is focusing upon moments, writes George Bell (1984) in his article "Poetry Therapy–A Focus on Moments," in *The Arts of Psychotherapy Vol 11*. Focusing on perceived reality and on what is happening in the present, he writes, fosters greater self-understanding. Writing in verse, he says, invites freedom, fresh insights, spontaneity, originality, creativity, and authenticity.

5. Poetry that activates the senses also activates memories, feelings, and a sense of beauty, wonder, and awe, writes Kenneth Gorelick in "Poetry on the Final Common Pathway of the Psychotherapies" (1989).

6. Gorelick (1989) establishes that poetry that draws upon the senses can activate buried memories and provide food for thought. It opens clients up to the outer world.

7. Koch's *Wishes, Lies, and Dreams* (1970), *Rose, Where Did You Get That Red?* (1973), and *Sleeping on the Wing* (1981) describe the author's experiences teaching poetry to children; *I Never Told Anybody* (1977) describes teaching poetry to a group of senior citizens in a nursing home. All books provide numerous specific examples of topics and activities that elicit responsiveness. His approach is not so didactic as it is one of helping members discover and present what they already possess.

8. An atmosphere in which all views are correct and acceptable fosters members' "social self," Gorelick (1989) writes. The capacity to communicate is enhanced as formulating and expressing viewpoints is the task of the members.

9. Gorelick (1989) writes that poetry promotes self-understanding: "By writing, the self is acknowledged and legitimatized. As spontaneous expressions of one's reactions are recorded, they are understood and taken in; one's internal world is changed. . . . Poems activate sensations, feelings, memories, as well as a sense of beauty, wonder, and awe." A group that composes collaborative group poetry instills in its members the need and the capacity to communicate and the need to manage conflicts. One discovers one's own responses through the exploration of others. All views are correct; all are acceptable. Each person has the task of formulating and sharing his or her viewpoint. The group must share the task of puzzling out meaning collaboratively. Group poems model the courage to think, to feel, and to take risks; they open up spontaneity and playfulness. Members create themselves through the group and in relation to it.

BIBLIOGRAPHY

I. Mental Illness

Arieti, S. *Creativity.* New York: Basic Books, 1976.
Arieti, S. *Understanding and Helping the Schizophrenic.* New York: Basic Books, 1979.
Arnheim, R. (1986) "The Artistry of Psychotics." *American Scientist.* Vol. 74 48-54.
Coles, R. *The Call of Stories.* Boston: Houghton Mifflin, 1989.
Jourard, S. (1964) *The Transparent Self.* New York: Wiley-Interscience.
Greene, R. R., and Ephross, P. H. *Human Behavior Theory and Social Work Practice.* New York: Aldine de Gruyter, 1991.
Laing, R. D. *The Politics of Experience.* New York: Ballantine Books, 1967.
Mann, N. A. et al. (1993) "Psychosocial Rehabilitation in Schizophrenia: Beginnings in Acute Hospitalization." *Archives in Psychiatric Nursing*, 7(3) 154-162.
Piercy, M. *Circles on the Water.* New York: Alfred A. Knopf, 1982.
Spotnitz, H. *Modern Psychoanalysis of the Schizophrenic Patient: Theory of the Technique*, 2nd Ed. New York: Human Sciences Press, 1985.
Ulman, E. et al. (1976) "The Mental Health Disciplines: Notes on the Development of 13 Disciplines That Play Important Roles in the Treatment of the Mentally Disabled." *Hospital and Community Psychiatry*, 27(7) 495-504.
Warner, R. et al. (1989) "Acceptance of the Mental Illness Label by Psychotic Patients: Effects on functioning." *American Journal of Orthopsychiatry*, 59(3) 398-409.
Winerip, M. *9 Highland Road.* New York: Pantheon Books, 1994.

II. Poetry and Creative Writing

Bell, G. L. (1984) "Poetry Therapy–A Focus on Moments." *The Arts in Psychotherapy.* Vol. 11 117-185.
Bowman, D. O. (1992) "Poetry Therapy in Counseling the Troubled Adolescent." *Journal of Poetry Therapy*, (6) 1 27-33.
Chase, K. "About Collaborative Poetry Writing," *Journal of Poetry Therapy*, 3 (2) 97-105.

Conrad, J. (1971) "The nigger of Narcissus." (Preface, p. viii) In *Three Great Tales*. New York: Vintage Books.

Gorelick, K. (1989) "Poetry on the Final Common Pathway of the Psychotherapies: Private Self, Social Self, Self-in-the-World." *Journal of Poetry Therapy*. 3 (1) 5-16.

Kaminsky, M. *What's Inside You, It Shines Out of You*. New York: Horizon Press, 1974.

Koch, K. *I Never Told Anybody*. New York: Random House, 1977.

Koch, K. *Rose, Where Did You Get That Red?* New York: Random House, 1973.

Koch, K., and Farrell, K. *Sleeping on the Wing: An Anthology of Modern Poetry with Essays on Reading and Writing*. New York: Vintage Books, 1981.

Koch, K. *Wishes, Lies, and Dreams: Teaching Children to Write Poetry*. New York: Harper and Row, 1970.

Kivnick, H. Q. & Erikson, J. M. (1983) "The Arts as Healing." *American Journal of Orthopsychiatry*. 53 (4) 602-618.

Mackey, R. and O'Brien, B. A. (1979) "The Use of Diaries with Experiential Groups," *Social Work with Groups*, Vol. 2, 175-180.

Mazza, N. and Price, B. D. "When Time Counts: Poetry and Music in Short-term Group Treatment." *Social Work with Groups*. 8 (2) 53-66.

May, R. *The Courage to Create*. New York: W. W. Norton & Co., 1975.

Myerhoff, B. *Number Our Days*. New York: Simon & Schuster, Inc., 1980.

Rossiter, C. (1992) "Commonalities Among the Creative Arts Therapies as a Basis for Research Collaboration." *Journal of Poetry Therapy*. 5 (4) 227-235.

Saltzman, J. *If You Can Talk, You Can Write*. New York: Warner Books, 1993.

Wadeson, H. (1981) "Self-Exploration and Integration Through Poetry Writing." *The Arts in Psychotherapy*. Vol. 8 225-236.

III. Social Group Work Practice

Brandler, S., and Roman, C. P. *Group Work: Skills and Strategies for Effective Interventions*. Binghamton, N.Y.: The Haworth Press, Inc., 1991.

Kurland, R. *Group Formation: A Guide to the Development of Successful Groups*. New York: United Neighborhood Centers of America, 1982.

Kurland, R. "Planning: The Neglected Component of Group Development," *Social Work with Groups*. Vol. 1, No. 2, Summer 1978, 173-178.

Kurland, R., and Salmon, R. "Self-Determination: Its Use and Misuse in Group Work Practice and Social Work Education," in D. Fike and B. Ritter (eds.) *Working from Strengths: The Essence of Group Work*. Miami, FL: Center for Group Work Studies, 1992, 105-121.

Northen, H. *Social Work with Groups*. New York: Columbia University Press, 1988.

Shulman, L. *The Skills of Helping Individuals and Groups*. Itasca, IL: F.E. Peacock Publishers, Inc., 1979.

Vinter, R. D. "Program Activities: An Analysis of Their Effects on Participant Behavior," *Individual Change Through Small Groups*, Glasser, Sarri, Vinter, eds., New York: The Free Press, 1974, 233-243.

She's Doing All the Talking,
So What's in It for Me?

(The Use of Time in Groups)

Dominique Moyse Steinberg

SUMMARY. This paper discusses the use of time in a group and suggests that practitioners conceptualize group time pluralistically rather than distributionally or linearly. Examples of each approach are presented and implications for practice are drawn. *[Article copies available for a fee from The Haworth Document Delivery Service: 1-800-HAWORTH. E-mail address: <docdelivery@haworthpress.com> Website: <http://www.HaworthPress.com> © 2005 by The Haworth Press, Inc. All rights reserved.]*

PROLOGUE

The other day, as I went over to help a small working group of students in my research class, I overheard their conversation, which went something like this . . .

Uh . . . who wants to go? I don't know. Do *you* want to go? I don't know–do *you* want to go? I don't know–do you want to go? I don't

Dominique Moyse Steinberg, DSW, is Adjunct Instructor at the Hunter College School of Social Work, 129 East 79 Street, New York, NY.

This paper was presented at Symposium XVII, Association for the Advancement of Social Work with Groups, San Diego, CA, October 1995.

This article was originally published in *Social Work with Groups*, Vol. 19 (2) © 1996 by The Haworth Press, Inc.

[Haworth co-indexing entry note]: "She's Doing All the Talking, So What's in It for Me? (The Use of Time in Groups)." Steinberg, Dominique Moyse. Co-published simultaneously in *Social Work with Groups* (The Haworth Press, Inc.) Vol. 28, No. 3/4, 2005, pp. 173-185; and: *A Quarter Century of Classics (1978-2004): Capturing the Theory, Practice, and Spirit of Social Work with Groups* (ed: Andrew Malekoff, and Roselle Kurland) The Haworth Press, Inc., 2005, pp. 173-185. Single or multiple copies of this article are available for a fee from The Haworth Document Delivery Service [1-800-HAWORTH, 9:00 a.m. - 5:00 p.m. (EST). E-mail address: docdelivery@haworthpress.com].

doi:10.1300/J009v28n03_12

know. Who *else* wants to go? *You* want to go? *I* don't care. Should *I* go? *You* go. *You* don't mind? No, I don't care. Okay . . . should *I* go . . . ?

Fortunately–for it was closing in on the end of class, someone finally "went!"

* * *

As humorous as this example is, more often than not this is the way people–including people who work with groups–tend to think about group time; and concerned with their ability to meet the needs of their members, groups often struggle with time management in just this way.

"How should we use our time together?" workers wonder. "How can everyone get their share?" "Should everyone get equal time?" "Should the one who needs it most get the most?" "How do we know who needs it most?"

Meanwhile, group members also wonder about group time. "When is it going to be *my* time?" they ask, and "If Miss X is doing so much talking, what's in it for *me*?"

* * *

After overhearing these endless "I don't knows" in class, I sat with the group; and while questions were asked and answered of the person who "went," I couldn't help but interrupt the process every few seconds to ask, "See how this applies to you, as well, Tom?" or "See how you need to do that too, Dick?" or "Isn't this basically the same issue you face, Harry?" I felt like I was working up a sweat, but the reward finally came, for as they began to discover their common ground, their heads began to bob in excitement and their pens began to "furiously" take notes.

* * *

INTRODUCTION

Generally speaking, the management of group time is guided by the assumption that whatever time one person "takes" or "gets" in the group is time that other group members will, in fact, have to "give" or "give up." And viewed in this way, that is, as a question of distribution, group time does indeed seem to pose an unresolvable dilemma.

The purpose of this discussion is to propose that rather than struggle with how to distribute time, practitioners shift the way they think about time. Just as in the song which says, "My time is your time, and your time is my time," this paper suggests that there is, in fact, always a multiple engagement of time in a mutual-aid system, no matter who seems to have the floor and that the most pressing practice question is less one of distribution than it is how a group gives any of its time whole-group meaning.

Time is central to social work with groups and to a great degree dictates the look and shape of a group. The passage of time has been offered as a paradigm for shaping expectations and interventions (see, for example, Berman-Rossi, 1992; Garland, Jones, and Kolodny, 1978; Glassman and Kates, 1983). The implications of time on pre-group planning and on goal-setting have also been explored at length (see, for example, Hartford, 1978; Kurland, 1978; Lowy, 1976; Northen, 1988), while some implications for using time also have been suggested by the literature on communication patterns and decision making (see, for example, Kurland and Salmon, 1992; Lowy, 1978; Middleman, 1978; Toseland, Rivas, and Chapman, 1984; Tropman, 1981, 1987).

However, even if it can be argued that at the broadest level all of the group work literature addresses time in one way or another, virtually none of it discusses the use of time with any specificity.

A NEW LOOK AT AN OLD PROBLEM

A number of strategies exist for managing time in groups, ranging from the "equal time for all" approach to the "squeaky wheel gets the grease" approach. The problem for practice is that none of the options which conceptualize time as a resource to be distributed in some manner are very satisfactory.

If time is distributed to group members in a so-called equal way, for example, how meaningful can content–particularly the talking type of content–be? Once we discount warm-up and ending time of even a 90-minute meeting, each of seven people is left with about ten minutes to call his or her own. Can any group, no matter how skilled the practitioner, truly do justice to any issue of importance in ten minutes?

On the other hand, if the "squeaky wheel" strategy is used to respond to competition for time, and if all the group members except the squeaky wheel think of themselves as being on hold or in "waiting" time for their turn, how can they help but feel like losers? Who knows if the group will ever get to "their" time or if their time will even come *in* time?

The following two excerpts illustrate this dilemma very clearly:

Excerpt One

Worker:	I would like to bring something up with the group. Some people have mentioned to me that there isn't always enough time for them to talk. Sometimes many people have pressing concerns, and we only have an hour and a half. I wonder if the group has ideas to deal with this problem.
June:	You are saying that for my benefit because I told you the other day.
Worker:	Yours and other people who mentioned it to me.
Gloria:	Well, I know I talked a lot when my daughter got in trouble but maybe the person who needs it most . . .
Worker:	How could we determine that?
Helen:	We could ask everyone, go around.
Claire:	Why don't you just pick?
Worker:	Well, I might on occasion, Claire. So, Helen mentioned going around. How so?
Claire:	Well, just ask who wants to talk, or each person says a little.
Worker:	Marie, what do you think about that?
Marie:	There's no way. The one who's most upset should talk.
Gloria:	Well, we'll just ask who wants to talk at the beginning.
Worker:	How will we help people who have trouble speaking up?
Claire:	I'm not sure. We'll ask around. I think we got a good idea, now.
Helen:	Yeah, we get the idea.
Worker:	Okay, we'll discuss it again and see how it is working out.

Excerpt Two (A Few Minutes of Silence)

Claire:	(giggles) Well, who's going to talk today?
Gloria:	I'm feeling really good. I had a good week. I'd like to listen to someone.
June:	Well, I had some trouble with this guy at school . . . uh, is it okay for me to talk? (addressing the question to the worker)
Worker:	Ask the group.
June:	What do you think? Does anyone else want to talk?

Helen: Well, I do a little, but you look really upset. I'll talk after.
Marie: Go ahead June, you look upset.

In this example, the group has identified three possible options for managing its time. One possibility is that the person who needs it most be the one to get it most. This solution only leads to another dilemma, however, which is how the group will determine which member does in fact need it most and by implication raises another question as well, which is what will happen to those who need it "less?"

In response to this new problem, the group identifies a second and rather novel option, which is that the worker might simply pick group members at his discretion. Clearly, the worker is not thrilled with this solution, as he glosses over it quickly on the way to other possibilities.

The group continues its discussion and eventually identifies a third possibility, which is that each person have the chance to talk in each meeting. As Claire puts it, perhaps each group member could "say a little."

In this example, two versions of "squeaky wheel" and one form of "equal time" have been identified as solutions to the group's time-management problem. But are these three options really the only ones available? The mutual-aid approach to practice would argue that no, they are not. It would claim that another option exists. It would argue, in fact, that practitioners need to adopt another approach to the use of time altogether. Only by adopting a *pluralistic* rather than distributive approach to the use of time, it would propose, can we help groups create mutual-aid opportunities; and only by helping the group's time become *filled* time for each and every group member, it would further argue, can we help groups actualize those opportunities.

What does it mean to have a pluralistic approach to time and to help group time become filled time for every group member?

First, developed as a paradigm for analyzing organizational systems (Whipp, 1994), a pluralistic approach to the use of time posits that systems function not through any linear action and reaction of their subsystems but through parallel processes. Time should be conceptualized not as a resource capable of being partialized or distributed, but must, instead, be understood in its original metaphysical form as a dimension, inescapably and invariably used by all things at once.

The way in which time is used may vary from thing to thing, of course, or in the case of groups, from person to person. We may even attach value judgments to how time is used. We may, for example, refer to time "taken" or time "spent" or time "wasted" or time "killed." In fact, we may even refer to "down" time. No matter how we judge the quality of its use, however, as a dimension, time does get used. Therefore, rather than think about the function of any system as a linear progression of its subsystems, it is more accurate to think about it as a reflection of simultaneous multiple activities.

To conceptualize time as a dimension and to adopt a pluralistic approach to its use also means (to borrow another concept, this time from economic theory) that time is always and automatically *fillable* (Owen, 1991). Filled time refers to time which is perceived as productive, while unfilled time refers to time which is perceived as wasted. If we perceive the use of time as being productive for us, then we perceive it as filled. If we perceive it as being *un*productive for us, then we perceive it as unfilled. In other words, whether or not *any* time is filled is always in the eye of the beholder, as it were.

Conceptualizing time in this way, then–in terms of being filled or unfilled–suggests that the most pressing practice question regarding group time is less one of giving any one group member "enough" time than it is one of helping group process provide filled time for the whole group. No longer is it "to fill or not to fill" for any one group member, but *how* to fill it for every group member *all* of the time.

If a group fills its time one member at time, as is often the case in the "presenter" scenario, for example, it is not unusual for group process to take on a one-way look; and it is not surprising that those group members who do not have the floor often feel as if their time is essentially unfilled. On the other hand, when a group fills its time with a search for mutuality–that is, when process takes on a two-way motion–then by providing an element of self-interest to each group member, the group has the potential to provide filled time for everyone in the group, not just the so-called presenter.

THE USE OF TIME TOWARD MUTUAL AID

Thinking about time as a dimension and capable of being perceived as filled or unfilled in plurality is particularly appropriate to helping groups engage in mutual aid. Take the case of Miss X, for example, who seems to be doing all the talking. Whatever type of group she is in, Miss X cannot help but do much of the talking as she describes her problem. And while Miss X may be using the time in a more *apparently* active way than are her fellow group members, they are never completely inactive. They must inevitably use this same time in some way. In some groups they may use it to listen to Miss X as would a polite audience. In others, they may use it to formulate advice. In some, they may even use it in a totally unrelated silent activity.

If mutual aid is to occur, however, when Miss X talks, her fellow group members must listen in a very specific way. They must listen with what might be called a self-referential ear (Kurland and Salmon, 1992). And while the group's process may *appear* to focus more on Miss X than it does on her fellow members because her situation is what catalyzed the discussion, this self-referential way of responding to and exploring Miss X's situation actually provides filled time for everyone in the group, as group members actively listen in order to clarify the issues, as they actively think about their own lives, and as they actively share the floor with Miss X by sharing and comparing stories and experiences. In short, as the members of Miss X's group think about their similarities, examine their differences, and explore the personal meaning of their similarities and differences, time becomes well spent, or "filled" for everyone in the group.

This use of time for *active* (i.e., *shared*) self-reflection in the service of self and others is crucial to mutual aid, because only through self reference can group members transform individual issues into their more generic form and as such make them useful to the whole group. In many approaches to the use of time in groups, on the other hand, the use of time begins and remains individually oriented. Time is used essentially to focus on and remain focused on the situation of the person who raises a problem or issue in the first place. In fact, even when group members are expected to learn by analogy, they are generally expected to do so in a quiet sort of way; for to actively share the floor with the person who initially "presented" would be perceived as infringing on that person's time.

No wonder problem-solving time in a group is so often perceived as predominantly other-directed and basically unfilled by those who did not raise the issue or immediate question.

A CASE IN POINT

Let us take the case of Miss X, and let us examine how a group goes about transforming individual time into filled time for everyone in the group.

While Miss X takes the time she needs to fully describe her situation, her fellow group members fill their time by helping Miss X better explain herself so that they can better understand what she means and what she feels. They interrupt her with comments like, "I don't understand what you mean." They ask for clarification with questions like, "Can you be more specific?" or "Can you think of an example?" And they ask for elaboration with questions like, "Can you say more about that?" In other words, as Miss X's co-members listen and react to what she is saying, they use their time to expand their understanding of the problem as Miss X describes it and to see the issues as Miss X sees them.

It may appear as if the group's focus is completely on Miss X at this point, because she is doing so much talking. Even now, however, time can be conceptualized as filled for all of the group's members as they actively help Miss X better define the specific issues to be addressed and identify the more generic issues to be understood.

It is here that the mutual-aid approach to individual problem solving parts company from most other approaches to that process (Kurland and Salmon, 1992, pp. 9-10). In many other approaches, group members are expected to make sense of the issues raised by Miss X primarily for her sake; and as a result, once they believe they understand Miss X's problem, they move directly into searching for solutions and advice for Miss X, even if they have found food for thought on their own behalf. In a mutual-aid process, on the other hand, group members are expected to use their listening time to make sense of the issues for their own sake as well as for the sake of Miss X. Even when group members think they see the issues as Miss X does, therefore, their exploration process continues, and it continues with a shift inward.

As group members come to believe that they see the issues as Miss X sees them, they ask themselves questions like, "Have I ever been in such a situation?" "What was it like?" "What happened for me?" "How did it make me feel?" They use their time, in other words, to reflect on the ways in which their own experiences, past and present, are similar to or different from those of Miss X. Some group members may recall similar situations and similar feelings. Others may recall similar situations but different feelings. Still others may recall similar feelings but different situations.

The exact scenario of similarities and differences does not really matter. What matters here is that by providing time for self reflection, time continues to be "well spent" not just for Miss X but for all the group's members.

Again, it might continue to seem as if the group's focus is only on Miss X because this self-reflection process is a silent one; but in fact, time can still be conceptualized as filled for all of the group's members as they begin to give the personal issues raised by Miss X whole-group meaning.

As group members think about their own lives and the ways in which their own experiences are like or unlike those of Miss X, they share their stories with one another. They bring to light some similarities. They bring to light some differences. And as the group seeks common ground, it explores the implications of its similarities and differences. Miss X's work of the moment is to use her life experience to inform and enlighten this process, while that of her fellow group members is to inform and enlighten it with theirs.

In other words, as their self-reflection process now becomes expressive, group members have an opportunity to deepen their understanding of themselves and their understanding of one another; and time continues to be filled for everyone in the group.

Once group members have shared their stories, the group does one of the things it does best: it brainstorms possible solutions to Miss X's problem. In their continued use of self-reference and self-reflection, group members revisit their own histories to contribute a variety of perspectives and possibilities for the group's view and review. "I remember when something like that happened to me," one group member might say, and go on to describe how the way in which he handled his own problem had worked out well. "I remember trying that too, but for me it didn't work so well," another might chime in and go on to share her own experience.

The group's focus may appear to shift back to Miss X at this point, as group members actively search for solutions to her problem. However, while they are thinking about her immediate needs, they are continuing to search their own experiences to find ways to be helpful.

Even as group members look for solutions to a so-called individual problem, therefore, it can still be proposed that time is filled for every group member as each one reflects on, and contributes his or her own skills and strengths to, the group's collective thinking process.

Eventually, as Miss X's fellow group members try to help her develop a course of action, the group's focus does shift back to her, as the group helps her make some plans for action specifically related to her situation. Nonetheless, even at this point, it can be said that time continues to be filled for the whole group, as everyone in the group has the opportunity to make personal meaning of what has been said and heard. In other words, as they think through the implications of Miss X's choices, they think about them on their own behalf as well with questions like, "What if I had . . . ?" or "What if I had to . . . ?" or "What if I were to . . . ?"

As group members talk about how the process of looking at Miss X's situation has contributed to their own ways of thinking, being, and doing, this process comes to a close. What began as individual time has become whole-group time, filled with mutual aid as all group members think about how they might address an old problem in a new light or how they might face a new problem with new resolve.

IMPLICATIONS FOR PRACTICE

There are several practice implications to thinking about group time as proposed here:

1. Moments in which one group member's issues appear to dominate must be conceptualized as windows of opportunity for mutual aid rather than as reflections of monopoly or "lopsided" group interaction.
2. Groups must be planned around strong commonality of need if we expect group members to use their time together to transform individual issues into collective food for thought. The stronger their commonality of need, the easier it will be for them to make such a transformation; the more abstract the commonality (e.g., "We all have human needs"), the more difficult it will be.
3. The group's purpose must be both clear and relevant if we expect group members to use their time together to reach common ground. If its purpose is either too vague or too loosely conceptualized (e.g., "The purpose of this group is to help people improve the quality of their life"), group members will have to reach *too* far to discover their common denominator.
4. Prospective or new group members must be educated about how the use of group time looks from a mutual-aid point of view, including how "individual" problem-solving time can be used to the group's advantage. We need to explain that mutual aid evolves not from equal presenting time but from using group time to explore and make personal meaning of so-called individual issues.
5. Expectations regarding the use of time must be included in the contracting process so that group members are prepared for the active pursuit of so-called individual issues rather than being left to wonder when it will be "their" time.

6. Whenever group members bring an issue to the group, this problem-solving approach must be initiated by asking them to talk more, not less. We must ask for information, seek closer scrutiny, greater clarification, and in such and other ways initiate the use of group time to give that issue the time it deserves. As we do this again and again, group members will come to learn that in the groups we have in mind, this kind of process is "normal."

7. Whenever the group evaluates its problem-solving process, group members must be helped to gauge the group's success by evaluating the quality of group time rather than the quantity of presentation time.

8. We must make particular use of those skills which help group members fill group time with two-way motion and which help group members identify common ground.

SUMMARY/CONCLUSION

In conclusion, traditional approaches to the use of time in a group may present more problems than they solve. Instead of approaching the use of time as something that group members have to "give" or "take," time should be conceptualized as inherently accessible to and inescapably used by each and every group member. Viewed in this way, then, the only practice question which remains with regard to its use is how to help the group create time "filled" for each group member *all* of the time.

Anyone who raises a personal issue in a group is bound to do much talking, since describing it fully requires stating, restating, explaining, elaborating, clarifying, and other forms of enlightenment. While this person is using group time to talk, however, the other group members must also make some use of that time; and while there may be different options for using that time, a mutual-aid process fills it with self-reference and self-reflection as group members seek understanding and mutuality.

Even if all group members cannot reach back to similar situations, they can think of situations, past or present, which have evoked similar feelings. In either case, once self reference is set in motion, group members have opportunities to clarify their own thinking, attitudes, and feelings at the same time that they seek to better understand those of others. They also have opportunities to reconfirm jobs well done, so to speak, to reexamine those perhaps not so well done, and to strengthen their resolve for new jobs yet to come. In short, they have an opportunity to contribute to thinking things through together in a personally meaningful way. Using time in this way is essential for helping a group develop and maintain mutual aid; it is what helps prevent, as Margaret Hartford coined it, "aggregational therapy" of individuals (1978, p. 23).

It is hoped that this discussion will encourage people who work with groups to review the way they think about and use time in their own work. Rethinking time as a dimension, adopting a pluralistic approach to its use, and helping so-called individual time become filled time for every group member all of the time can improve our practice by permitting us to focus our attention on quality rather than quantity. If we remain preoccupied with the "distribution" of time, we will inevitably use our *own* time anxiously awaiting those "interruptible" moments instead of using our time to help the group discover mutual aid.

SELECTED BIBLIOGRAPHY

Berman-Rossi, T. "Empowering Groups Through Understanding Stages of Group Development," in *Social Work with Groups*, 1992, Vol. 15, Nos. 2/3, pp. 239- 255.

Dewey, J. *How We Think*, Boston: Heath, 1910.

Garland, J., Jones, H. E., and Kolodny, R. L. "A Model for Stages of Development in Social Work Groups," in *Explorations in Group Work*, Saul Bernstein, ed. Hebron, Ct.: Practitioner's Press, 1978.

Glassman, U., and Kates, L. "Authority Themes and Worker-Group Transactions: Additional Dimensions to the Stages of Group Development," in *Social Work with Groups*, 1983, Vol. 6, No. 2, pp. 33-52.

Hartford, M. "Groups in the Human Services: Some Facts and Fancies," in *Social Work with Groups*, 1978, Vol. 1, No. 1, pp. 1-10.

Kurland, R. "Planning: The Neglected Component of Group Development," in *Social Work with Groups*, 1978, Vol. 1, No. 2, pp. 173-178.

Kurland, R., and Salmon, R. "Group Work vs. Casework in a Group: Principles and Implications for Teaching and Practice," in *Social Work with Groups*, 1992, Vol. 15, No. 4, pp. 3-14.

Lowy, L. "Decision-Making and Group Work," in *Explorations in Group Work*, Saul Bernstein, ed. Hebron, CT: Practitioner's Press, 1978.

_____. "Goal Formulation in Social Work with Groups," in *Further Explorations in Group Work*, Saul Bernstein, ed. Boston, MA: Charles River Books, 1976.

Middleman, R. "Returning Group Process to Group Work," in *Social Work with Groups*, 1978, Vol. 1 No. 1, pp. 15-26.

Northen, H. *Social Work with Groups*. New York: Columbia University Press, 1988.

Owen, A. "Time and Time Again: Implications of Time Perception Theory," in *Lifestyles: Family and Economic Issues*, 1991, Vol. 12, No. 4, pp. 345-359.

Shulman, L. *The Skills of Helping Individuals and Groups.* Itasca, IL: F. E. Peacock Publishers, Inc., 1984.

Toseland, R., Rivas, R. F., and Chapman, D. "An Evaluation of Decision Making Methods in Task Groups," in *Social Work*, 1984, Vol. 29, pp. 339-347.

Tropman, J. E. *Effective Meetings: Improving Group Decision Making.* Beverly Hills, CA: Sage Publications, 1981.

_____. "Effective Meetings: Some Provisional Rules and Needed Research," in *Social Work with Groups*, 1987, Vol. 10, No. 2, pp. 41-55.

Whipp, R. "A Time to be Concerned: A Position Paper on Time and Management," in *Time and Society*, 1994, Vol. 3, No. 1, pp. 99-116.

The Personal in the Political: Exploring the Group Work Continuum from Individual to Social Change Goals

Marcia B. Cohen
Audrey Mullender

SUMMARY. This article analyzes three examples of group work practice in order to examine the relationship between internal and external change goals across the practice continuum. Using the conceptual framework of the British model of self-directed group work, the authors explore the potential of social action groups to meet individual, interpersonal, and social needs. The three practice illustrations include a poetry group in a service center for homeless and low-income adults, a peer support group in a recipient-directed mental health agency, and a community meeting group in a homeless shelter. *[Article copies available for a fee from The Haworth Document Delivery Service: 1-800-HAWORTH. E-mail address: <docdelivery@haworthpress.com> Website: <http://www.HaworthPress.com> © 2005 by The Haworth Press, Inc. All rights reserved.]*

KEYWORDS. Group typologies, social action, social change, self-directed group work

Marcia B. Cohen, PhD, is Associate Professor at University of New England School of Social Work, Hills Beach Road, Biddeford, ME, USA (E-mail: mcohen@mailbox.une.edu). Audrey Mullender is Professor, University of Warwick Department of Applied Social Sciences, Warwick, England, UK (E-mail: assar@csv.warwick.ac.uk).

This article was originally published in *Social Work with Groups*, Vol. 22 (1) © 1999 by The Haworth Press, Inc.

[Haworth co-indexing entry note]: "The Personal in the Political: Exploring the Group Work Continuum from Individual to Social Change Goals." Cohen, Marcia B., and Audrey Mullender. Co-published simultaneously in *Social Work with Groups* (The Haworth Press, Inc.) Vol. 28, No. 3/4, 2005, pp. 187-204; and: *A Quarter Century of Classics (1978-2004): Capturing the Theory, Practice, and Spirit of Social Work with Groups* (ed: Andrew Malekoff, and Roselle Kurland) The Haworth Press, Inc., 2005, pp. 187-204. Single or multiple copies of this article are available for a fee from The Haworth Document Delivery Service [1-800-HAWORTH, 9:00 a.m. - 5:00 p.m. (EST). E-mail address: docdelivery@haworthpress.com].

Available online at http://www.haworthpress.com/web/SWG
© 2005 by The Haworth Press, Inc. All rights reserved.
doi:10.1300/J009v28n03_13

Group work has been described as falling in the middle of the social work practice continuum. The literature on generalist social work practice conceptualizes group work as *mezzo* level work, falling in between *micro* (individual and family change) oriented interventions on one end and *macro* (community and social change) oriented intervention on the other (Parsons, Hernandez, and Jorgensen, 1988). There is a long history of debate within social work as to the relative importance of different parts of the continuum (Bisno, 1956; Cloward and Epstein, 1965; Lee, 1930; Schorr, 1959; Specht and Courtney, 1994), with individual change and societal change framed as dichotomous goals.

There is a parallel continuum within social group work, ranging from the remedial model, emphasizing individual change, to the social goals model, emphasizing social change. Falling between them is the interactional model, emphasizing mutual aid and interpersonal growth. All three represent abstract conceptualizations of group work associated with particular theoretical traditions (Toseland and Rivas, 1998). In practice, however, group models are not necessarily so systematically ordered. If we blow up the photograph to a larger size, a finer grain appears which reveals that many groups actually represent an overlap of approaches. For example, a remedial model psychotherapy group may incorporate an educational component, use skill building activities, and foster mutual aid. Similarly, a social action group might use program activities and encourage the development of mutual support among group members.

This article will explore the relationship of group work models to "real world" group practice. It may be that the theoretical models, as currently articulated, fail to do justice to the "fine grain" of actual group work practice. Workers may use techniques and styles eclectically, in response to changing member needs, rather than maintaining a rigid allegiance to a single model. This non-partisan approach would certainly be in keeping with Wood and Middleman's (1989) principle of "following the demands of the client task" (p. 35) and Breton's (1995) caution against workers preempting the direction of group work by pigeonholing groups through a taxonomy of models. This interpretation raises several questions, however. Does this flexible approach lead to the models becoming blurred beyond recognition? And, alternatively, do broad models remain clearly discernible in practice, with groups moving along a continuum of models, changing focus as dictated by the needs of the group?

Before probing these issues further using several group examples, a brief overview of the traditional models of group work will provide contextual grounding for our discussion.

THE REMEDIAL MODEL

The over-arching goal of remedial model group work has been described as restoring and rehabilitating individuals who are "suffering from some form of social maladaptation," (Papell and Rothman, 1966, p. 71) or "behaving dysfunctionally" (Toseland and Rivas, 1995, p. 53). The authors most often associated with the remedial model include Garvin (1987), Vinter (1974) and Yalom (1985).

Members of remedial groups have individual treatment plans, generated and executed by the worker (usually a group therapist), which determine their goals within the group context (Reid, 1991). Papell and Rothman describe the worker-determined, individual treatment goal as the "central and most powerful concept" in remedial group work (1966, p. 72). Remedial groups are highly leader-directed with the therapist actively intervening in and managing group processes. Vinter (1974) describes multiple roles for the remedial group leader, including: functioning as the object of member identification and drives, acting as the agent of group-legitimate norms and values; defining individual tasks and goals, and controlling members' roles in the group.

THE INTERACTIONAL MODEL

The primary goal of interactional group work is the development of a mutual aid system among group members. Often referred to as the mutual aid model, it is associated with a number of theorists, most notably Schwartz (1961) and Gitterman and Shulman (1994). Interactional group work incorporates some of the remedial model's concerns with individual change, but has as its primary focus the interpersonal dimension of group work. The group worker in the interactional model is seen as having two clients, the individual group member and the group as a whole (Schwartz, 1961; Shulman, 1992). A primary role of the worker is to mediate between these clients, "search(ing) out the common ground between the individual and the group" (Schwartz, 1961, p. 21). Another important worker role is facilitating the development of mutual aid as it unfolds within the group (Shulman, 1992).

THE SOCIAL GOALS MODEL

The social goals model has roots in the settlement house tradition and in the social movements of the 1960s (Papell and Rothman, 1966). Referred to in more recent literature as social action group work, the central goals of this model are social change and the empowerment of oppressed populations. Proponents of empowerment-oriented approaches to social action group work include: Breton (1995), Cohen (1994), Cox (1991), Gutierrez and Ortega (1991), Lee (1994), and Mullender and Ward (1991).

The role of the worker in this model is less directive (though no less active) than in the other two models. This is consistent with the emphasis on empowerment, which has been defined as "having the choice to participate in the decisions that affect one's life, and the life of one's society and community" (Breton, 1994, p. 27). The role of social action group workers includes facilitating opportunities for the empowerment of group members, assisting group members with the process of determining social action goals and strategies, and challenging internal and external forms of oppression.

Over 30 years ago, Papell and Rothman (1966) pointed to a lack of adequate theoretical underpinnings in the social goals model. Since that time, a sound theoretical framework for social action groups has been developed which integrates feminist and empowerment practice theories with the century old social action tradition in social group work. As Lee (1994) describes, an array of empowerment-oriented approaches to social action group work emerged in the 1980s and 1990s, in North and South America, France, and Britain.

SELF-DIRECTED GROUP WORK

One of the most fully developed of the empowerment-oriented social action approaches is the British model of self-directed group work. Formulated by Mullender and Ward (1985, 1991), self-directed group work targets external goals identified by group members through a process which involves them in focusing, in turn, on *what* are the major problems in their lives, *why* these exist, and *how* to tackle them. A notable feature of the approach is a clear value-base which is outlined in the form of six practice principles emphasizing: the avoidance of labels, the rights of group members, basing intervention on a power analysis, assisting people to attain collective power through coming together in groups, opposing oppression through practice, and group workers facilitating rather than leading (Mullender and Ward, 1991).

Inherent in these values is an assumption of a social structural analysis of the issues facing marginalized groups. Self-directed groups do not have therapeutic purposes. Indeed, the groups seek to challenge the fact that group members may have become, or could potentially become, negatively labeled as a result of interventions that inappropriately seek change at the individual or family level, rather than working to empower the group to tackle wider injustices. Intrapersonal and interpersonal change may, however, come about as a consequence of participation in self-directed groups.

One critique of the self-directed model (Norwegian group work educator, Ilse Espelund, personal communication) is the limited attention paid to the affective content of group process, something which is bound to be a major factor in the functioning of even the most task-oriented and sociopolitically aware groups. Revisiting and re-analyzing the self-directed group work model may help to explore where, and to what extent, personal and interpersonal issues might be addressed within groups primarily focused on social change goals. It might be that a single group work model can span a larger section of the group work continuum than has hitherto been suggested, without blurring the defining features which distinguish it as being predominantly one kind of group or another.

Group work is, after all, a fertile, living medium whose exponents continually develop fresh responses to the challenges they encounter in practice. It would be unrealistic to suppose that all that has been published about groups, to date, fully represents all that has been actually achieved in group work practice. Group workers in the "real world" are in the vanguard of creativity and innovation. Researchers and theorists have the arguably less difficult task of observing, analyzing, and making sense out of what happens in practice. Conceptual taxonomies have their place in advancing our understanding of group work practice but they may of necessity be rather bald generalizations. It is valuable to revisit and refine them periodically to insure that they remain reflective of the realities of practice.

We offer three practice illustrations as a point of departure in our exploration of the group work continuum. Our primary emphasis will be on examining the relationship between the observed groups and the theoretical model of self-directed group work. We hope that this inquiry will shed light on the connections between the affective content and mutual aid function inherent in all groups and their specific role in social action groups. In particular, we will demonstrate that all three levels of involvement (personal, interpersonal, and social) can be present in groups that might be assumed to be working at just one level. From these practice examples, we will draw the inference that the traditional categorization of groups fails to capture their complexity and recognize that these categories are not necessarily mutually exclusive. Finally, we will draw on social work theory to explain the unique properties of social action groups which enable them to incorporate personal, interpersonal, and social change concerns.

THE POETRY GROUP

A poetry group at an agency serving homeless people was the practice example which first suggested to us that remedial, interactional, and social goals models were not necessarily mutually exclusive. The Poetry Group appeared to be working at all three levels. This was a group with explicit social action aims which also celebrated and worked on feelings and relationships.

This group has been described as having " . . . the following mutually agreed on goals: to meet weekly to write together, to organize poetry readings for the public, (and) to educate the public and to counter negative stereotypes about homeless people by giving voice to their experiences . . . " (Cohen and Johnson, 1997, p. 134). These goals reflected members' interests in creativity and self-expression as well as community action. While framed as a self-directed group, weekly group meetings consisted of writing individual and group poems. The group's more external focus was realized at periodic poetry readings which were open to the public. The group facilitator and many of the group members saw poetry readings as critical opportunities for educating the wider community about the realities of severe poverty. This goal was not uniformly shared within the group, however. Some of the participants at weekly group meetings were drawn to participate solely out of a desire to write and receive feedback on their work. Others attended because the group was a warm and welcoming place where they received support and encouragement. In practice, the group's external and internal goals were not dichotomized.

The Poetry Group was developed as a self-directed group and the facilitator consciously sought to embody Mullender and Ward's six practice principles. The group incorporated a conscious social structural analysis which can be discerned in some of its poetry, for example:

Billy

When Billy turned five and started school the teacher asked,
"What do you want to be when you grow up?"
And these are the things that Billy didn't say:
"I want to be a junky and a dope addict.
I want to get married too young and beat my children and my wife.
I want to sell my body to perverts in the park
for twenty bucks or crack cocaine.
I want to live on welfare, food stamps
and be a burden to my fellow man.
I want to beg for quarters
so I can buy some beer.
I want to sleep under bridges
and have young punks call me bum
I want to stay in shelters
and slowly go insane.
I want to drink cheap wine
and puke and piss my pants.
I want to eat in dumpsters and soup kitchens
and smoke cigarettes that I find.
I want to be called lazy and shunned
by so-called gentlemen.
I want to smell of unwashed skin
and grow to hate my fellow man.
I want someone to kill me for the things I've become.
I want to be called a vagrant and a bum.
The things that Billy did say
are irrelevant because he's dead.
Killed by the hero of the town ("Zeek," as quoted in Cohen and Johnson, 1997, pp. 136-7).

Group readings of poems such as *Billy* generated powerful discussions about the oppressive nature of homelessness, the rights of poor people to full participation in their community, and the need to educate members of the public with class privilege about the realities of life in the streets. The group's social change focus coupled with the worker's clarity about her role as group facilitator and consultant, rather than group leader, establishes this group as self-directed in orientation. Although the medium through which the group worked was that of an activity group, and some members were drawn by the activities rather than the broader social action objectives, the social goals level was clearly present in the group and had been mutually agreed to and actively pursued by group members.

The group was externally focused, with a goal of community education. At the same time, it carried both individual and mutual aid elements in that members had a weekly opportunity to explore their own internal creativity in the company of like-minded individuals. Whereas there can be social goals in a group accompanied by individual growth and mutual support, the converse is rarely true of groups developed with the primary intention of achieving individual change or mutual aid. Indeed, it is quite unusual for a therapy or support group to incorporate social change goals. In contrast, a group working towards social change inevitably achieves individual growth as a by-product of its work. Not only do groups aimed solely at individual change fail to achieve social goals, they sometimes serve to "keep the lid on" social problems by helping people feel a little better about adverse situations rather than seeking to change them.

This group example confirms Mullender and Ward's (1989) contention that the personal benefits for members of self-directed groups are considerable. The proponents of self-directed groups may appear to understate the importance of intrapersonal and interpersonal processes, due to the model's strong emphasis on groups' external agendas. In fact, internal group dynamics in self-directed groups are as rich as in any group.

The creative energy, the engagement with feelings, and the development of mutual support through writing about painful experiences were all important elements of the Poetry Group's process. They served to revitalize rather than distract from the externally focused activity of the group. Because the group worked on so many levels at once, members were able to take different things from it at different times. This fits Breton's (1994) observation that "Good empowerment work . . . requires that all levels of work, the personal, interpersonal, and structural/political, be addressed" (p. 31). At its core, however, the Poetry Group remains a self-directed group with lessons to teach us about the affective content of such groups. Though anger and despair are writ large in the poetry and were evident in the group's discussions, the members did more than get in touch with and support each other through these emotions. The group moved into an enthusiasm for struggle and pursuit of social change, *taking control* of their own group goals and *taking action* toward meeting those goals.

THE PEER SUPPORT GROUP

This second example, like the first, demonstrates that the same group can have the potential to combine all three levels; personal, interpersonal, and social. But, in this case, the group members themselves decided not to work on social goals. The example is an important one because the organizational context of the group was highly conducive to pursuing social action aims. There was a radical feel about the setting, far more, in some ways, than the Poetry Group. Placing the two examples side by side points up the importance of looking into the heart of what a group is actually working on, its stated purpose, and what level of change members have signed up for.

The host agency in this example was a recipient-directed mental health organization with historic ties to the mental patients' liberation movement (Chamberlin, 1978). The setting itself incorporated Mullender and Ward's (1991) six practice principles: consciously avoiding the labeling of its members, emphasizing members' rights, promoting a conscious awareness of power relationships within the mental health system, advocating social action aimed at gaining collective power, and actively opposing oppression. In this sense, the agency operated as a self-directed group, with a strong board of directors composed of democratically elected service recipients exercising collective power in agency decision making. Service recipients, as board members and committee members, were in charge of all personnel decisions (hiring, firing, raises, promotions, etc.) which had the effect of transforming power relationships between service providers (staff) and recipients (members).

The Peer Support Group was developed and facilitated by a social work student. It was framed as a group where service recipients would provide support and mutual aid to each other in relation to personal and interpersonal issues of daily life. The worker saw her role to be primarily one of facilitating the development of a mutual aid system among members of the group. She had, in fact, as an agency staff member, responded to the request of several service recipients to begin a support group. The choice of the name "Peer Support Group" was intentional. The group purpose was, from the outset, related to the promotion of mutual aid. The group's name also conveyed the student's understanding that she was not responsible for providing support in the group, rather that her role was to assist the group in developing its own internal support mechanism. The group was planned as a time-limited, 10-week group, with the goal of providing a forum for members to share day-to-day concerns within a climate of mutual aid. Most group meetings focused on problem solving and peer support around personal and interpersonal issues such as relationship difficulties, family problems, and dilemmas related to coping with disabilities.

It would have been unlikely for a group planned and designed in this fashion to work towards external change goals. Although broader societal issues, such as the oppression experienced by people in the mental health system, were raised in the group, these were discussed at the level of how the individuals who raised them might personally deal with them, rather than as shared issues to be tackled collectively. In effect, such a broadening of focus had been ruled out from the start by the short term nature of the group as well as by its name and stated focus. Members themselves had not expressed interest in an externally directed, activist focus, either when requesting the group or while participating in it.

The Peer Support Group did have some potential to develop into a social action-oriented group. Members occasionally raised and discussed issues of social injustice. One member, for example, talked about being stigmatized because of his psychiatric history. The group began (using Mullender and Ward's three questions) to talk about *What* was the problem–discriminatory attitudes in the mental health system and in society–and even touched on *Why* this problem exists–a medical model that individualizes and pathologizes mental distress. They did not, however, move as a group into owning this analysis as something around which they wanted to take action. They did not work on *How* it might be tackled. Social change interests might have emerged had there been more time for group members to explore their common experiences. This would probably have necessitated moving beyond straight discussion into the use of group work techniques that emphasize the *Why* question and help the group analyze its own response in a way that raises collective consciousness (Mullender and Ward, 1991).

This analysis reveals that the Peer Support Group, although member-directed, did not set externally focused, social goals. It had the defining features of a mutual aid group, with explicit interactional goals, rather than the defining characteristics of a social action group. This example provides useful clarification of the criteria for self-directed group work, as well as reflecting some of the richness of the interactional model. It also demonstrates that mutual aid groups can operate effectively within a context of awareness of social injustice and oppression.

THE COMMUNITY MEETING

This third example, in contrast to the second, is one where social change goals were given such a high profile that, traditionally, the personal and interpersonal content of the group would have gone unnoticed. Yet, they were clearly present and important to the group. The Community Meeting was organized as a weekly forum for service recipients at a homeless day shelter. Its explicit purpose was to increase recipient input into decision making within the host agency. The community meeting format was developed by two agency social workers who believed that the staff should share their decision making power with service recipients. Despite some initial resistance from other staff members (see Cohen, 1994), the group was successful in gaining a power base within the agency. Service recipients welcomed the opportunity to have a voice in agency decision making. The group facilitators helped members to set their own direction and goals. Over time, group members became secure in their ownership of the group and increasingly comfortable with the workers' nondirective, consultative roles. The community meeting achieved one of its original goals during its second year, the creation of two recipient seats on the agency's board of directors. A proposal for recipient inclusion had been soundly defeated prior to the community meeting group's inception. Community meeting members had advocated long and hard for direct representation on the board and had begun attending and participating in open board meetings even prior to the change in policy. Board members' perceptions of recipients improved as a result of increased social contact and they were finally swayed to include recipients on the board, albeit in a limited fashion.

The Community Meeting would appear to meet the criteria of a self-directed group, in terms of following the model's six practice principles and having an external focus rather than one which assessed members' life struggles as requiring therapeutic intervention focused on individual concerns. The group also demonstrated the potential of repeating the *What, Why, and How* steps of the model in further cycles, through naming, analyzing, and taking action on fresh problems when members began to voice broader structural concerns beyond the boundaries of the host agency. The organizational focus for change had been external to group members; the subsequent concerns went wider still, into issues such as the shortage of affordable housing, the stigmatizing and discriminating tendencies of the social service system, and the punitive nature of the city's workfare program. The group began to tackle this latter issue but quickly discovered that the public officials who administered the system were immune to their arguments. This led the group to analyze the force of structural barriers erected against them, including the societal labeling of them as the problem, while recognizing that the restructuring of patterns of work and welfare is a global issue requiring large scale changes.

The Community Meeting was undeniably a self-directed group within a social action tradition. Its purpose and goals were externally focused and were set collectively by group members. Any individual gains by group members were serendipitous; they were not the key purpose for which the group was established. Although a strong mutual aid system emerged amongst members, and was encouraged by the workers, this internal support mechanism was secondary to the group's more activist goals. Mutual aid functioned in the service of these goals; in times of frustration and discouragement it was the glue that held the group together. Similarly, the group's attention to its own affective process was critical to the group's survival. For example, when Gabby, one of the group's original members, announced that he would be leaving town, the group initially was devastated. Gabby was a warm and charismatic man who had played a crucial leadership role in the group. Group members, with the support of the facilitators, were able to communicate their feelings of anger and love toward Gabby, openly expressing emotions of pain and abandonment. This uncensored process helped the group to renew their commitment to each other and to their shared goals, allowing them to move forward after Gabby's departure.

Mutual aid and affective expression were not the group's defining features, however. This was a radical, politicized group, characterized by and proud of its collective understanding and activism. It provides an excellent example of the multiple levels on which an effective group operates, with all that this implies for group facilitator awareness and skills.

DISCUSSION

All group members, whatever type of group they join, face personal and interpersonal issues in their lives–heavily labeled and oppressed people perhaps more than most. All groups, even self-directed groups, are bound to face personal and interpersonal issues because they are composed of human beings in struggle, whose pain and anger are brought to the surface in an inescapable way. The choice of collective action as a response to the struggle puts each group member in connection with others who offer shared understanding and mutual support.

A self-directed group does not tip over into being an interactional group just because it deals with interpersonal material or a remedial group because it deals with personal content. These elements, however, may be far more important to the functioning of the group than has generally been recognized in the social action literature. Conversely, there may be interactional groups, like the Peer Support Group described above, which despite a social structural analysis in the mind of the group worker and some preliminary discussion of societal issues in the group, never direct themselves towards external change goals. These groups do not fit the model of self-directed group work (Mullender and Ward, 1991), even where the group members have primary responsibility for the direction of the group.

The fact that we can detect varying degrees of individual, interpersonal, and socially-directed aspects in a range of groups, suggests two things. First, there may be more richness and potential in any one model than may be readily apparent, a possibility which lends itself to fruitful exploration. Secondly, Breton (1995) is correct in her suggestion that an overly-rigid taxonomy of group work models, which does not allow for this co-existence of levels within any one group, may be harmful, and may mean that the worker risks blocking the group from healthy development along a range of different levels.

This does not imply, however, that there are not distinguishable models within group work, nor that these cannot be represented diagrammatically. What it does mean is that rather than the familiar continuum of three mutually exclusive levels of operation: *personal, interpersonal, and social,* we might better reflect the complex world of practice if we think in terms of all groups having individual content, most groups valuing and utilizing mutually supportive interactional content, but only some groups reaching out beyond their own boundaries towards an external social change focus. We might diagram the range of group work models as follows:

Model	Focus of Goals	Content
Remedial	therapeutic	individual
Interactional	mutual aid	individual + interpersonal
Social Goals*	social change	individual + interpersonal + social
*includes self-directed and all other social action groups		

In this reformulation, the defining features of the three types of groups are quite clear. Although they do not have mutually exclusive content or concerns, remedial groups seek change *solely* at the individual level while, at the other end of the continuum, social goals groups are the *only* ones to pursue social change goals. Interactional groups occupy the middle ground of the continuum, where they are primarily focused on fostering interpersonal growth and the development of mutual aid systems.

Our analysis has demonstrated that social action groups have far more individual and interactional content than has been suggested in the literature. They can potentially span the entire continuum of levels of operation, from the intensely personal to the outwardly political. The same level of individual need might, in some cases, be met by any of these three types of groups but only the group with social change goals will meet it primarily by helping the person understand the wider structural causes behind the distress. Further work is needed to clarify which forms of personal distress are so internally caused (rather than internally experienced) that it would be irrelevant to respond to them at a combined individual/interactional/social level.

THE ROLE OF THEORY

The above formulation does not address the theoretical underpinnings that lead the group worker to favor one kind of group over another. It is inaccurate to assume that groups of different types are always established to address very different kinds of problems. A recipient of psychiatric services, for example, might just as readily be referred to a psychodynamic psychotherapy group at an outpatient clinic, a self-help group at a drop-in center, or a social action group at a mental health advocacy project. The biggest difference between these groups does not reside in the group members, who may have similar kinds of distress, be at similar points in their psychiatric careers, and be experiencing similar problems in their lives. Rather, the key variable here is the theoretical orientation of the group worker who chooses to facilitate a particular type of group because of a particular belief system regarding the causes of that distress, that psychiatric career, and those problems. The worker's theoretical biases are usually buttressed by the ideology of the particular practice setting.

What can be said about the theories espoused by workers in self-directed and other social action groups that lead them to choose these models? Crucially, these are theories which deal with issues of oppression and empowerment (see, for example, Freire, 1972). An understanding of these theories reveals why self-directed and other social action groups work on so many levels. Thompson (1992), for example, illustrates how oppression and discrimination always operate simultaneously at personal, cultural, and societal levels. From this theoretical perspective, it follows that a self-directed group would span personal, interpersonal, and social elements of change.

Thompson's model is one of anti-discriminatory practice which rightfully challenges social workers to challenge the social injustices they encounter in themselves and their working environments. We can go further, however. Being empowered implies more than an absence of oppression. Within each area of oppression, there are now strengths-based theories which place the standpoint of the oppressed group at the center–making it the world view, rather than a deviation from a powerful norm. Some examples of such theories are feminism (Jordan, Kaplan, Miller, Stiver and Surrey, 1991), the African-centered paradigm (Graham, 1999), lesbian theory (Gonda, 1998) and the social model of disability (Oliver, 1993). None of these perspectives is internally uncontested but each turns the world on its head by arguing that the hitherto dominant view does not equate with all available knowledge; rather, that new knowledge needs to be generated from new vantage points by asking new questions of previously silenced people. This is of immediate relevance to group work since it challenges notions of who owns the group's knowledge and understanding, as well as its goals.

The richest literature on *how* oppressed and silenced people can generate their own knowledge is that of participatory action research (PAR). PAR has three key elements which can inform our quest for what is specific to groups with socially directed goals. These three elements are *participation*, *action*, and *education*, in the sense of consciousness raising, which forms an essential bridge between the first two elements. It can take the form of participatory action groups taking on community issues, as has happened, for example, in Colombia (de Roux, 1991), or women's issues in India (Mies, 1991), or Aboriginal Canada (Match International, 1990). To achieve participatory action, group members and facilitators learn together and collectively generate new understanding, working as equals in this process.

PAR has a time-honored history on a global scale that illustrates what achievements are possible when people work together for change. In Western-style group work practice, the setting of social action goals similarly flows from involving group members as full partners in analyzing and understanding their own problems. Thus, it is not just social change goals which make self-directed and other empowerment groups distinctive, it is the theory and process through which these goals are arrived at. This is always a *participatory* process and an *active* style of group work, based on a social structural analysis. Self-directed group work and PAR owe equal allegiance to Freirian theory. They simply apply it in different settings and often on a different scale, though for overlapping purposes.

CONCLUSION

The quest for democratically rooted understanding and collectively organized change was discernible in both the Poetry Group and the Community Meeting examples discussed above. The Peer Support Group traveled a similar road, and achieved some useful structural insights, but did not go the full journey toward social action based on collectively generated understanding. All three of these groups tell us something more about the external focus that makes self-directed groups distinctive. They also tell us what self-directed groups share with all other groups: the individuality of human experience at times of pain and distress and the resilience of the human spirit in fortifying others to survive that experience. These aspects of externally-oriented groups have not always been fully acknowledged or explored in sufficient depth. Having recognized that they are present in all groups, the challenge will be to appreciate their strength without diverting attention (in analysis or in practice) from broader goals of social change. We hope that our exploration of the group work continuum and the unique characteristics of self-directed groups will lead to further dialogue and practice-based analysis.

REFERENCES

Bisno, H. (1956). How social will social work be? *Social Work*, 1(2), 12-18.
Breton, M. (1994). On the meaning of empowerment and empowerment-oriented social work practice, *Social Work with Groups*, 17(3), 23-35.
Breton, M. (1995). The potential for social action in groups. *Social Work with Groups*, 18(2/3), 5-13.

Chamberlin, J. (1978). *On Our Own: Patient-Controlled Alternatives to the Mental Health System*. New York: McGraw-Hill.

Cloward, R.A. and Epstein, I. (1965). Private welfare's disengagement from the poor. In Meyer Zald (editor), *Social Welfare Institutions*. New York: Wiley.

Cohen, M.B. (1994). Who wants to chair the meeting? Group development and leadership patterns in a community action group of homeless people. *Social Work with Groups*, 17(1/2), 81-87.

Cohen, M.B. and Johnson, J. (1997). Poetry in Motion: A Self-Directed Community Group for Homeless People, in Jeanne Gill and Joan Parry (editors), *From Prevention to Wellness Through Group Work*. New York: The Haworth Press, Inc., 131-142.

Cox, E.O. (1991). The critical role of social action in empowerment oriented groups. *Social Work with Groups*. 14(3/4), 77-90.

de Roux, G.I. (1991). Together against the computer: PAR and the struggle of Afro-Colombians for public service, in O. Fals-Borda and M.A. Rahman (editors), *Action and Knowledge: Breaking the Monopoly with Participatory-Action Research*, New York: Apex Press.

Freire, P. (1972). *Pedagogy of the Oppressed*. Hammondsworth: Penguin Press.

Garvin, C. (1987). *Contemporary Group Work*. Englewood Cliffs, NJ: Prentice-Hall.

Gonda, C. (1998). Lesbian theory, in S. Jackson and J. Jones (editors), *Contemporary Feminist Theories*. Edinburgh: Edinburgh University Press.

Gitterman, A. and Shulman, L. (1994). Mutual Aid Groups, Vulnerable Populations, and the Life Cycle. New York: Columbia University Press.

Graham, M.J. (1999). The African centered worldview: Developing a paradigm for social work, British Journal of Social Work.

Gutierrez, L. M., and Ortega, R. (1991). Developing methods to empower Latinos: The importance of groups. *Social Work with Groups*, 14(2), 23-43.

Jordan, J.V., Kaplan, A.G., Miller, J. B., Stiver, I. P. and Surrey. J. L. (editors) 1991. *Women's growth in connection: Writings from the Stone Center*. NY: The Guildford Press.

Lee, J.A.B. (1994). *The Empowerment Approach to Social Work Practice*. NYC: Columbia.

Lee, P.R. (1930). Social work: Cause and function. *Proceedings of the National Conference of Social Work, 1929*, 3-20.

Match International Centre (1990). *Linking Women's Global Struggles to End Violence*. Ottawa, Ontario Match International Centre.

Mies, M. (1991). Women's research or feminist research? The debate surrounding feminist science and methodology. In M.M. Fonow and J.A. Cook (editors), *Beyond Methodology: Feminist Scholarship as Lived Research*. Bloomington and Indianapolis: Indiana U. Press.

Mullender, A. and Ward, D. (1985). Towards an alternative model of social groupwork. *British Journal of Social Work*, 15, 155-172.

Mullender, A. and Ward, D. (1989). Gaining strength together. *Social Work Today*, 20(50), 14-15.

Mullender, A. and Ward, D. (1991). *Self-Directed Groupwork: Users Take Action for Empowerment*. London: Whiting and Birch.

Mullender, A. and Ward, D. (1993). The role of the consultant in self-directed group work. An approach to supporting social action in Britain. *Social Work with Groups*, 16(4), 57-79.

Oliver, M. (1993). *Social Work: Disabled People and the Disabling Environment.* London: Jessica Kingsley.

Papell, C. and Rothman, B. (1966). Social group work models: Possession and heritage. *Journal of Education for Social Work*, 2, 66-77.

Parsons, R.J., Hernandez, S.H., and Jorgensen, J.D. (1988). "Integrated practice: A framework for problem-solving." *Social Work*, 33, 417-421.

Reid, K.E. (1991). *Social Work Practice with Groups: A Clinical Perspective.* Belmont, CA: Brooks-Cole Publishing.

Schorr, A. (1959). The retreat to the technician. *Social Work*, 4(1), 29-33.

Schwartz, W. (1961). The social worker in the group. In *New Perspectives on Services to Groups.* New York: The National Association of Social Workers, 7.

Shulman, L. (1992). *Skills of Helping Individuals, Families and Groups*, Third Edition, Itasca, Il.: Peacock Publishers, Inc.

Specht, H. and Courtney, M. (1994). *Unfaithful Angels: How Social Work Has Abandoned Its Mission.* New York: The Free Press.

Thompson, N. (1998). *Anti-Discriminatory Practice* (second edition). Basingstoke: Macmillan.

Toseland, R. and Rivas, R. (1998). *Introduction to Group Work Practice*, Boston: Allyn and Bacon.

Vinter, R. (1974). The essential components of social group work practice. In Glasser, Sarri and Vinter (editors), *Individual Change Through Small Groups*. NY: The Free Press, 9-33.

Wood, G. and Middleman, R. (1989). *The Structural Approach to Direct Practice in Social Work*, New York: Columbia University Press.

Yalom, I.D. (1985). *The theory and practice of group psychotherapy,* New York: Basic Books.

The Use of Purpose
in On-Going Activity Groups:
A Framework
for Maximizing the Therapeutic Impact

Whitney Wright

SUMMARY. This article explores the purposeful use of on-going activity in social group work. It examines the ways in which the group's purposes fluctuate over the group's life, with the activity-oriented purpose taking precedence in beginnings, the personal growth-oriented purpose taking precedence in the middle stage, and both purposes sharing importance in endings. Throughout the paper, illustrations from a co-ed teen ceramics group are provided. *[Article copies available for a fee from The Haworth Document Delivery Service: 1-800-HAWORTH. E-mail address: <docdelivery@haworthpress.com> Website: <http://www.HaworthPress.com> © 2005 by The Haworth Press, Inc. All rights reserved.]*

KEYWORDS. Activity groups, programming, group purpose, stages of group development

Whitney Wright, CSW, is Youth Specialist at the Family Center, 66 Reade Street, New York, NY 10007.

This article was originally published in *Social Work with Groups*, Vol. 22 (2/3) © 1999 by The Haworth Press, Inc.

[Haworth co-indexing entry note]: "The Use of Purpose in On-Going Activity Groups: A Framework for Maximizing the Therapeutic Impact." Wright, Whitney. Co-published simultaneously in *Social Work with Groups* (The Haworth Press, Inc.) Vol. 28, No. 3/4, 2005, pp. 205-227; and: *A Quarter Century of Classics (1978-2004): Capturing the Theory, Practice, and Spirit of Social Work with Groups* (ed: Andrew Malekoff, and Roselle Kurland) The Haworth Press, Inc., 2005, pp. 205-227. Single or multiple copies of this article are available for a fee from The Haworth Document Delivery Service [1-800-HAWORTH, 9:00 a.m. - 5:00 p.m. (EST). E-mail address: docdelivery@haworthpress.com].

doi:10.1300/J009v28n03_14

Two very experienced social group workers recently led a painting group at a clinic for adolescents with HIV. They wanted "a break" from the heavy talking groups they were used to leading. For the first session, they decided to have the kids trace the outlines of their bodies on long rolls of paper. The members were then given various colors of paint to decorate their images. The members showed discomfort in the closeness of the tracing process, but went along with the activity. When it was time to fill in the bodies, they surprised the leaders with their reactions. One member left it blank and said she had nothing inside. Another put Xs over his eyes and said he was already dead. Another drew a skull and cross-bones for a face. Another took the back of the paint brush and ripped up his outline. The members made fun of each other's paintings and even ruined a few of them. The group met one more time where just two members returned. It never met again.

This example shows the power of activity and demonstrates its potential misuse. The following pages explore the purposeful use of on-going activity in social group work. The article looks at effective means to harness long-term activities in order to maximize their clinical impact on a group. How Purpose fluctuates with the developmental stages of the group will be addressed. A framework for social group workers is provided.

GROUP DEVELOPMENT

A distinct process takes place from which a cohesive and dynamic group burgeons from a mere assembly of individuals. The members' interaction changes as the group progresses. Over time, the group becomes a means for the members to make positive changes in their lives and to grow individually and as a group. Though every group is distinct and special, each one has a life cycle that follows a pattern of stages. The stages in social group work are the identifiable behavior patterns occurring at certain points along the span of group development.

Stages of group development have been a hallmark in social group work theory for decades. The extensive literature on group development (see, for example, Garland, Jones, Kolodny, 1973; Northen, 1988; Schwartz, 1976; Toseland and Rivas, 1998; Garvin, 1997; Glassman and Kates, 1990; Brown, 1991; Henry, 1992) demonstrates the importance of group stage in selecting appropriate interventions. It is these interventions that assist the group in developing into a microcosm able to achieve its given purposes.

Since Bruce Tuckman's seminal work, "Development Sequence in Small Groups" (1965), and Garland, Jones and Kolodny's "A Model for Stages of Development in Social Work Groups" (1973), many authors have built their own interpretation of group development in social group work. The breakdown of stages varies in specificity. Sub-phases even emerge within major stages. Whether the theory denotes three stages or seven, and regardless of the date of publication, each one follows a basic framework found in all groups (Schwartz, 1976; Toseland and Rivas, 1984; Garvin, 1997). For the purposes of this paper, three stages–Beginnings, Middles, and Endings–will be used.

The beginning stage of group development is marked by fear, anxiety, and ambivalence in the members about what is to come. Members may want to embrace the group, but are afraid of rejection and failure. The group leader needs to assist each member's entry into the group. The middle stage is the bulk of the group's life cycle. As members settle into the group, overcome ambivalence, and begin to feel more comfortable, they become more emotionally invested in the group. Individual differences are recognized: roles and status are defined. Members are able to struggle, assist each other, and focus on the work of the group. The ending stage of a group cycle is characterized by openness and free and easy communication. On the other hand, it also elicits feelings of anxiety and ambivalence about terminating the group. Regression, denial, and hostility often come to the surface. It is a time for the members to stabilize the gains they have made, evaluate the group experience, reminisce, and look ahead to new experiences (Kurland, 1999).

ACTIVITY GROUPS

As humans we express ourselves through many mediums and interact using our whole body. Therefore, to dichotomize "talking" and "doing" is misleading (Shulman, 1971). In group work with activities, verbalization is an integral and equally important component of the "doing" experience. Activities are used with the understanding that personal growth comes not merely from mastering an experience or skill, but also from the cognitive recognition of the complexity of that experience.

When we speak of "activity" or "programming" in social group work, we typically refer to the purposefully chosen game, exercise, or project, often lasting no longer than the duration of one session. Programming also refers to the long-term use of a single activity–such as art, dance, writing, or sports–that continues for the duration of the group's life cycle. This paper will assume the latter in its discussion of activity-based group work.

The recognition of the potential benefit of programming in social group work dates back to some of the discipline's earliest scholars (Boyd, 1938; Coyle, 1947; Wilson and Ryland, 1949). In fact, the early preoccupation with programming may have thwarted the acceptance of group work as a theoretically and clinically sound method into the greater discipline of social work (Middleman, 1968). Even today, many group work practitioners misunderstand the use of activity. Many downplay the programming component or avoid it entirely in fear that their groups may not be considered serious or clinical, despite the extensive literature on its therapeutic value.

Ruth Middleman solidified programming as a method in group work practice through the publication of her notable and influential book, *The Non-Verbal Method in Working with Groups* (1968). More recently, the numerous advantages of the use of programming have been well explored in group work literature. Programming provides an alternative means of encouraging verbal expression, influencing members' behavior, and assisting individuals and the group in their progression towards achievement of group purpose. Fundamentally, members can express themselves creatively and non-verbally through the use of programming.

Activity-oriented content can be used to serve a range of purposes in a group. Helen Northen (1988) outlines many of the values of activity groups. The stimulation of verbal communication of feelings, the facilitation of problem solving, the development of relationships, and the enhancing of self-esteem through skill mastery emerge as values pervasive in much of the literature on activity-oriented group experiences (Whittaker, 1974; Brandler and Roman, 1991; Malekoff, 1997).

The value of the use of activity is evident in the extensive theoretical literature. Similarly, the applicability of activity-oriented group work to divergent populations has also been documented by many practitioners working in the field with their own groups. For example, Erica Schnekenburger (1995) illustrates the value of a writing group for mentally ill adults. Dromi and Krampf (1986) use board games as a means towards emotional growth with maladaptive Israeli adolescent boys. George Getzel (1983) examines the use of the arts in social group work through a poetry group with the elderly. Melvin Delgado (1983) discusses the value of activity for treating Hispanic adults. And Andrew Malekoff, in his book *Group Work with Adolescents; Practice and*

Principles (1997), explores at length the appropriateness of the use of activities with young people. Clearly, a substantial body of activity-centered literature illuminates the diverse application and value of activity groups in social group work.

PURPOSE IN ACTIVITY GROUPS

Just as a plethora of literature exists purporting the importance of activities in social group work, a voluminous body of literature also maintains the importance of Purpose in social group work. But Purpose remains nebulous far too frequently in practice, regardless of the undeniable emphasis in the literature on the need for clarity of purpose (see, for example, Toseland and Rivas, 1998; Kurland and Salmon, 1998a; Garvin, 1997; Henry, 1992; Brown, 1991; Glassman and Hates, 1990; Northen, 1988). Clarity of purpose in a group is often an overlooked component of group planning (Kurland, 1978; Kurland and Salmon, 1998a). Often, practitioners are unable to give a clear explanation of the purpose of their own groups. Likewise, when members are asked: "What is the purpose of your group?" one can be met with an array of unclear answers.

Purpose is that ultimate goal for which the group has formed. It is the collective expectation the group is striving to achieve. It is the destination to which the leader is helping the members arrive. Purpose includes the goals and objectives of the group that have been developed based on the need of the population served. Though members may have their own ideas about how those objectives play out in their own lives–their own personal goals to be realized through their membership–Group Purpose is the same for the whole group. It needs to be clear, concise, understood, and ascribed to by the group members.

Purpose in on-going activity groups can be even further misunderstood. Instead of conceptualizing the mastery of an activity as a purpose in itself as well as a tool to reach a more personally-centered goal, often the activity becomes the sole purpose of the group. Often in an activity group, it is unclear how the group differs from a drawing class, a basketball class, a drama class, a sewing class. Mastering the activity certainly needs to be a purpose of the group. But it is the aspect of personal or community growth that makes the activity group a social work group. Therefore, dual purposes need to coexist in activity groups. For example, adolescent boys' mastery of the skill of carpentry may be the activity-centered purpose in a group, while increasing impulse control may be the personal growth purpose. It is how each purpose is played out over the group's life cycle that fosters a greater therapeutic impact of the group.

As each stage of group development carries its own indicative behaviors and needs of the members, program comes with corresponding elements. Each phase dictates the type of activity appropriate for the members at that particular time (Ross and Bernstein, 1976; Brockway, 1999). For example, an activity centered around sharing intimate secrets would not be appropriate to use in the beginning stage of a group. Robert Vinter (1974) developed activity-setting dimensions to consider in selecting group activities. Though his dimensions were devised for short-term activities, they can be applied to the purposeful use of one on-going activity in a group. Vinter's activity-setting dimensions will be used in the following analysis of the purposeful use of activity in social group work. A ceramics group with fourteen-year-old boys and girls from a community based agency in Brooklyn, New York is drawn upon for examples. The purposes of the group were mastery of the medium of ceramics and increased self-understanding.

BEGINNINGS

"What is this group all about?" "Will I be able to accomplish the task?" "Who is this leader?" "Can I trust her?" "Will I fit in?" These are all typical feelings in the mind of a member walking into the first group session. New members want closeness with the leader and the other members. They want to show who they are and to be accepted by the group. They want to understand why they are there. They want to know that they will be able to accomplish that purpose.

The work of the group at this stage is made complex and trying because of the flip side of these wonderful and inquisitive desires. For as much as new group members may want to embrace the group head-on and share themselves, they can be terrified of the repercussions of doing so. They don't know if what they share will remain private. They don't know if other members will like what they bring to the group. They don't know what will be asked of them in the following sessions. All of these fears often keep group members from fully engaging in the beginning stage of the group. They may explore but retain a right to draw back when they feel vulnerable. In other words, for almost every approach, there comes an avoidance.

First and foremost, the members need to be oriented to the group. The purposes of the group need to be explained in full to the group as a whole (even if purpose was covered individually in pre-group contacts). Since it may be unclear to the members how purpose will actually play out in the group, it needs to be discussed, agreed upon, and accepted. At this point, purpose will most likely remain elusive for the members for a number of sessions. The worker needs to continue to check in with the group to make sure all are in agreement as to why they are a part of the group.

The group is now forming. It is defining itself–molding into its own entity with its own norms, values, and patterns of communication. Cohesion allows for the group to shape itself. And commonalities among the members are the glue that fixes that cohesion in place. The beginning stage sets a tone for the life cycle of the group to come.

As explained above, Purpose in activities groups is divided into at least two parts. Members most often come to an activity group for the activity-oriented purpose (the art, sport, etc.). Few people will come to a dance group if they don't like dancing, or a painting group if they don't like art. But they may stay for the personal growth purpose (e.g., increased self-esteem, the building of community, problem-solving, etc.). Moreover, in the beginning stage, it can be difficult for the members to understand the personal growth purpose. Therefore, the activity-centered purpose is accentuated in the beginning stage of development. The emphasis on the activity-centered purpose provides structure for the members in order to assuage their anxiety and help them enter the group.

The particular use of the activity needs to be geared to beginning stage needs of the group members. High worker control in deciding how the activity is used provides a safe environment where the members do not need to take risks. Rather, they have the direction, structure and approval they need at this uneasy time. They may have fear that they will not be able to master the medium or that other members will be better than they. Low skill demand, low prescriptiveness (the quantity of rules or complexity of instructions), and low competitiveness will allay members' insecurities regarding the medium and their ability to accomplish the task at hand. Anxiety about not being accepted into the group can be managed by structuring the activity so that all members work at the same competence level, regardless of the prior skills of some members. As the group moves into middles, the skill level will begin to diversify. At this point members do not yet feel accepted into the group. The activity's emphasis on commonalities will work to connect the members and facilitate that process of acceptance.

The activity also needs to enable group norms to begin to be set. Everyone working together, acceptance of each member's participation, and helping each other are all norms important in social group work. For example, a baking group may begin with everyone making yeast bread together. Each member's participation is important so that all the ingredients are added and mixed thoroughly. Each member can then get the same amount of dough and make their own loaf, thus allowing them to become comfortable with the baking process while not being asked to produce it all on their own. The similar quality of their loaves will help bring superficial yet crucial commonalities to the surface. This purposeful use of the activity orients them to the group by fostering cohesiveness.

The members may exhibit ambivalence or even aversion towards the activity, especially those who have never attempted it before. Members' attitudes towards the activity can be an indication to the worker of their comfort level with the activity and in the group. High worker controls, high individual assistance, and low skill demand help mitigate the fear of the activity.

The following example illustrates a member's attitude about the activity and how it functioned as a barometer of their ease with the activity and in the group. This excerpt is from the first session of the co-ed teen ceramics group. Introductions, contracting, and a thorough discussion of Purpose and members' expectations of the group had taken place. Basic instruction in pinch method had been covered, including a demonstration by the worker. All members were given the same amount of clay and were making basic pinch bowls.

James: This clay smells gross and it's getting all over my hands. Eww, disgusting–can I go wash my hands?

Worker: You're right. It smells gross if you aren't used to it. Does anyone know what it is made of?

Tyrone: Dirt.

Worker: Right. And we're not really used to smelling dirt. But think you'll get used to it pretty soon. (Worker models smelling it up close and not being bothered by it.) And you are also right, James, that it gets all over our hands. I sort of want to wash mine, too. But if we try to keep our hands clean, then we won't really be able to mold the clay. Messy hands is just part of ceramics. I promise you it's not permanent. (Worker holds up a molded hunk of clay and models very messy hands. She walks over to him to help him start his bowl.)

Jessica: What if you have an itch?

Michael: Use the back of your hand.

The worker smiles at the suggestion and models using the back of her hand to scratch her nose. James nods and trepidaciously sticks his thumb into his hunk of clay.

Here James is expressing his discomfort in the group and desire to leave and "wash his hands" (of the group). His fuss about the clay reflects his need for assistance in entering the group. The worker's individual assistance as well as her modeling of comfort with the medium provide the support necessary for a member to approach the activity and join the group.

The following excerpt again illustrates the need for high worker controls. It also illuminates how commonalities play a vital role in the beginning stage. The members were having a difficult time maintaining an ideal wetness and thickness of their pots and controlling the pressure of their fingers on the clay. Jessica pushed too hard and broke through the edge of her bowl.

Jessica: Oh, I ruined it. I broke the side of my bowl. I hate this. I can't do this.

Worker: It looks to me like something other than a bowl now. Can anyone think of what it looks like?

Tyrone: It looks sort of like a pitcher.

Worker: That's exactly what I was thinking.

Jessica's face lit up. She turned it into a pitcher. Two other members turned their bowls into pitchers, too.

Since the activity-oriented purpose is emphasized in the beginning stage, neither example included deeper connections to members' feelings in the group or life outside the group. If these two excerpts had been taken from the middle stage of the group, James's difficulty engaging in new experiences or his feelings of being left out of the group may have been explored. Likewise, a discussion of the benefit to looking at potential positive outcomes of mistakes might have been prompted by Jessica's pitcher.

MIDDLES

As the group begins to move from the beginning to the middle stage of development, members are still unsure of exactly where they fit into the mix. Struggles for power, status, and role definition are characteristic of this transition. Exploring and testing of the situation and of the worker still take place. But once they enter the middle stage, members have a better sense of their place in the group. The similarities among the members that were so important in beginnings fall away to the recognition and appreciation of differences. The group as an entity begins to become meaningful, as do members' own personal goals. They can feel more comfortable sharing intimate information about themselves, their feelings, their history, their struggles, their opinions. Risks of self exposure, which once seemed inconceivable in the beginning of the group, now come more freely. Such risks enable mutual aid to take place: Members work on problems openly and help each other. Efforts to do so are lauded and encouraged by other members. Throughout the middle stage, the group becomes valued as a unique and special experience.

The focus on the activity in beginnings builds a safe environment for the work of the group to eventually happen. As the members begin to deepen their investment in the group, the personal-growth purpose emerges as more central than before. The members are able to focus their discussion on issues important in their lives. Though the activity remains an integral part in the group, it is used in different ways than in beginnings and plays a secondary role to the personal-growth purpose. Purpose needs to be periodically addressed and used as a reference point for the group.

The worker initiated controls in beginnings shift to the members in middles. They have more freedom to choose how they will use the activity and can put it aside at their own will. A higher minimum competence level permits risk-taking with the activity. As members express themselves individually through the activity, the differences among them are highlighted. The members become comfortable in the roles they play in the group and are ready to take personal risks in verbal discussion. The activity can now be used to initiate verbal discussion that demands problem solving, mutual aid, self expression, or self examination. For example, a weight lifting group that may have started with everyone lifting the same amount and learning how to do it properly, may move on to each person deciding on how and why they want get in shape. The individualized increased weight capacity or more demanding exercises could initiate group discussion about challenging your self, body image issues, femininity versus masculinity, anger management, etc. (depending on the group's personal-growth purpose).

The following excerpt illustrates how the activity can ease the members into deeper discussion in the beginning of the middle stage. It exemplifies their ability to start to connect the activity to their lives, to open up and take risks, to see differences among themselves, and to challenge themselves and the group. The activity is still a pivotal part of the discussion, but the more personally-centered purpose is burgeoning.

Everyone had kept at least two clay pieces to be fired except James. He was frustrated at his limited ability to form the clay. The rest of the group was moving on to more advanced pieces but he was still stuck. He began to smash his clay with the rolling pin.

James: I'm never going to be left back in school. I'm too smart for that. That's for stupid people.

Rhonda: You don't have to be stupid to be left back.

James: Yes you do and I'm not stupid.

Worker: I think James may be voicing something that others of you could be feeling. Everyone works at a different pace and is comfortable with different skills. Each of you is moving along at a different pace with your clay projects. Seeing other people's projects could make someone feel left behind by the group.

Jessica: Michael is going really fast.

Michael: (Shrugs his shoulders) I think it's fun.

Worker: So what if everyone had to go as fast as Michael?

Rhonda: We wouldn't do a very good job.

James: It wouldn't look like that (he points to a dog that Michael was working on).

Worker: So it can sometimes be a good thing to go at a slower pace, even to stay back a year in school.

Rhonda: I stayed behind last year.

Worker: What was it like for you?

Rhonda: It was a lot better. I felt like I could do things better.

The following example illustrates how norms are set in place by the middle stage (in this case, helping each other). The individual expression through the activity facilitates an appreciation of differences. A continued assessment of Purpose throughout the life cycle of the group conditions the members to consider what the group is about on an on-going basis.

Tyrone: Your mask looks like Wolf Man.

Rhonda: I wanted to make something scary.

James: That's some scary shit all right (he was helping Rhonda make her mask because he already finished his). Mine is more like a Martian, and look at Theresa's cat (Theresa smiles).

Worker: What would make you want to have a scary mask?

Rhonda: To scare people.

Worker: Who do you want to scare?

Rhonda: I could scare all those people on the street.

Tyrone: Yeah, there are crackheads all over my neighborhood. They bump into me all the time. I just want to . . . (he smashes a piece of clay with his fist).

Rhonda: Yeah, you have to pretend you're really tough so they don't mess with you.

Tyrone:	If someone seems mean, you don't want them to mess with you. You have to show them you're not gonna take it.
Worker:	How do you show them?
Tyrone:	I just give people a look or I say something tough.
James:	Yeah, you have to show them that you can be mean, too.
Theresa:	I wear this blue bandana, the Crips, you know.
Tyrone:	But I'm not like that all the time. Sometimes I'm really nice on the street. I help old ladies or women with their babies.
Worker:	It makes me think of our masks.
Tyrone:	Yeah (he laughs in recognition of the metaphor) like sometimes we have nice masks on and sometimes we have mean ones on.
Rhonda:	I can be different in different places. It's like I have different me's.
Worker:	What brings out each you?
Rhonda:	It's 'cause the way people make me feel I should be.
Tyrone:	I don't think this group is just about clay anymore.

The discussion continued along the lines of how the purpose of the group is shifting. We then continued to explore how the members need to change–or put on different masks–depending on where they are and what is demanded of them (i.e., home, school, in the ghetto, with their counselor, in the group, etc.).

By the time the group fully enters the middle stage, norms are well established. The members understand and find meaning in the growth-oriented purpose. The activity initiates verbal discussion that may not otherwise take place. Learning from the experience and expanding it to life outside the group comes more naturally for the members. The activity then holds increased emotional investment because it is imbued with deeper meaning. The following example illustrates how the activity is used in middles to access the growth-oriented purpose.

There had been some discussion of the members' discontent with their individual counseling. Rhonda was making a fist to symbolize how she felt about her counseling relationship. Jessica had complained about not trusting her counselor.

Jessica:	This looks bad (she smashes her clay bunny on the table).
Worker:	Jessica, I've been noticing a pattern of yours. I think you get frustrated that your project doesn't look like you want it to right away so you smash it.
Jessica:	But it didn't look good.
Worker:	I know it can be hard to put a lot of time and patience into something until it looks like you envision it.
Jessica:	Yeah, it's too hard.
Worker:	What other times have you guys found it hard to be patient and stick with something until it's how you want it to be?
Rhonda:	I've been working on this fist for weeks. It's still not how I want it. I almost smashed it a bunch of times but I didn't.
Worker:	What helped you keep from smashing it?
Rhonda:	I just kept thinking about the effort I had put into it. Jessica, just keep thinking about a bunny.
Worker:	This is reminding me of the struggles some of you are having with your relationships with your counselors.
Jessica:	I want to quit counseling. She doesn't understand.
Worker:	It can take time and patience to build a relationship until it finally looks the way you want it to–just like it takes time and patience for that hunk of clay to look like a bunny.
Jessica:	But I want to quit counseling (she smashes the bunny on the table).

Michael: You are just making it harder for yourself. Now you have to keep making the same thing over and over again.

Worker: So I'm hearing you say that in the long run it is harder to keep smashing things or quitting than to commit yourself to it.

Rhonda: It is easier at first, but then it's worse. Your counselor might really be able to help you.

Tyrone: And your rabbit could turn out good.

The activity continues to initiate discussion throughout Middles but is secondary in importance to the self-growth purpose. The discussion is the focus of the group. Members can exercise self determination by putting the activity aside and do so at will. The final excerpt from the middle stage illustrates how the activity is still present but no longer the emphasized Purpose.

Tyrone had been working on the same slab bowl for about four sessions. Several sessions passed where he sat with it in front of him, participated in the group discussion, but barely touched it at all.

Tyrone: I don't want to do this anymore. Maybe I'll smash it.

Worker: Do you want to smash it?

Tyrone: No. I want you to finish it for me.

Worker: What makes you want me to do it?

Tyrone: Because it takes too long and I don't have enough time. I have too much homework. Our teachers give us way too much to do at home. But it really doesn't matter because I get my mom or my sister to do it. They just do it for me 'cause they can do it a lot faster.

Worker: So you are asking me to do the same thing that your mom and sister do for you.

Tyrone: I just can't finish it. Look at all those cracks.

Worker: It sounds like when you get overwhelmed with something you give it over to someone else to do for you.

Tyrone:	Yeah, I guess so. Okay, I don't even want to finish it. I'll just throw it away. I just don't want to deal with it.
Worker:	You are frustrated by finishing this bowl and it's become a block for you. (Tyrone nodded.) Has anyone else been blocked by finishing something and wanted to throw the whole thing away?
Rhonda:	It's like that with my poetry.
Worker:	How?
Rhonda:	Sometimes I can't think of an end to it. I get frustrated and throw the whole thing away.
Worker:	What is it like to think about the poems you have thrown away?
Rhonda:	I wish I had them. I wish I had just finished them.
Worker:	Can you think of what kept you from finishing them?
Rhonda:	I just got stuck. All I had to do was one line but I couldn't.
Worker:	I see a theme of throwing everything away instead of facing the struggle and frustration of getting over the hump. It's sort of like repeating grades and how hard it can be to finish so you can pass. Does anyone want to share what it was like when they were trying to finish a school year that you then had to repeat?
Tyrone:	I'm doing the ninth grade over.
Worker:	Can you remember what it was like when you were trying to finish it the first time?
Tyrone:	I just got bored and didn't go to class. I could have passed but I just stopped going at the end.
Michael:	Just like Rhonda's poetry.

The discussion continued to address inability to deal with frustration and feelings of being overwhelmed and how it can result in self sabotage in school and in personal relationships. Several members mentioned pretending their problems didn't exist so they didn't have to deal with them.

Worker: I hear that a lot of you guys pretend there's no problem so you don't have to face whatever it is.

Rhonda: Yeah. Sometimes that's easier than looking at what's going on.

Tyrone: I haven't told anyone, but my brother tried to stab my mom last week. The cops came and everything. I just stayed in the other room watching TV. I pretended like it wasn't even happening.

James: Yeah. It's different when it's your family. It hurts more.

This initiated a discussion about domestic violence in the members' families and how they have coped with it. Each member joined in on their own with a story to tell. Other members supported those who had a difficult time talking about it. Two of the members cried. Theresa, who did not speak very much in the group, gave tissues.

ENDINGS

All too often the delicate nature of the termination stage in groups is neglected by practitioners. It is a very fragile but critical stage for the members. It concludes the group's life for them and allows them to incorporate the experience into their relationships in the future. The members need to make sense of what their experience in the group has meant to them. They need to revisit and rethink different parts of the group's cycle. The ending stage is a time of reminiscence, review, and evaluation.

Though communication comes freely by this stage, termination can elicit feelings of anxiety and ambivalence about ending the group. Members need to be able to express their feelings about ending and abandonment (by the group and the leader). Members need to talk about changes that have been made in themselves and the group. High worker initiated controls in the activity will help provide members with stability as their involvement in the group begins to wane. Individualized minimum competence level helps them put closure on their experience while not adding new challenges that they may not be able to meet in the little time remaining. Involvement of the whole group can help the members express deep feelings symbolically, to stabilize gains made, and to reminisce.

As the ending stage approaches, the activity oriented purpose and the personal growth purpose become more balanced. Both need to be discussed as separate and connected group purposes and evaluated. The activity may have to take precedence over discussion if remaining time is limited and a product needs to be completed. The activity needs to be structured so that the discussion stimulated can be easily linked to issues of termination. The activity needs to unite the group in their efforts to put closure on their experience.

Examples of appropriate uses of activities for the ending stage include preparing a final dinner in a cooking group, producing a final performance in a dance or drama group, or creating a mural in a painting group. The chosen final use of clay in the ceramics group was a collage that all members and the leader could contribute to. The final excerpt illustrates how a final activity can help the members through the difficult transition out of the group.

The worker chose a collage for the final project. It would let each member contribute at his or her own skill level but still produce something together. It enabled much of what needs to take place in endings to happen. The worker explained the collage as the final termination project. What to do with the collage had not yet been discussed.

Worker:	Everyone can add what they want to the collage.
Michael:	I want to make a house to put on it.
Worker:	What does a house mean to you?
Michael:	Safety.
Worker:	So this group has been a safe place?
Rhonda:	Yes.
Worker:	Has it always been?
Jessica:	No not always, sometimes it wasn't safe.
Worker:	When wasn't it safe?

The group discussed times when they didn't trust each other and what happened in the group to help them gain each other's trust.

Jessica: I'm gonna write trust on the collage because it was important here. Maybe we can write trust and safety in the house you're making.

Tyrone: I'm just doing this dot. That's it.

Worker: You don't want to add anything else?

Tyrone: I don't feel like it.

Worker: This needs to be completed today so we can glaze it next week. So what we've put together at 5:30 is what the collage will look like.

Tyrone: What's the point? The group's ending anyway.

We discussed how people felt about not meeting anymore, both the advantages and the disadvantages. Members expressed how they became close with each other, how they liked helping each other and being helped, and how much they will miss the group.

Rhonda: Well, I'm putting this heart on it so she'll remember me.

Michael: That's good because you made a lot of hearts.

Worker: You guys think I'm going to forget you.

Tyrone: Yeah.

Theresa: I think so, too.

Worker: What makes you think I'll forget you?

Theresa: 'Cause you're the leader.

Tyrone: And you have lots of groups.

Rhonda: But this one's different and we want you to remember it.

Jessica: Let's all make our first initials and put them on the collage.

Rhonda: Then we can give the collage to her so she'll have part of everyone in the group. Tyrone, do you want me to make your "T" for you?

Tyrone: No that's okay, I'll do it.

CONCLUSION

Practitioners need to embrace activity-oriented group work as complex, organized, and deeply clinical. Social group work with activities is not about the activity itself, but rather how that activity is used over the life cycle of the group (see Figure 1). Groups change and grow over time, as do their purposes. Purposes in activity groups need to flow with the natural development of the group, filling the changing needs of its members through the progress of the group. The structured framework provided here (see Figure 2) in which to use on-going activities will allow social group workers to more fully understand the potential impact of activities on the members. It can guide the group worker to help enable an activity group's therapeutic possibilities to flourish.

FIGURE 1. How Emphasis of Purpose Fluctuates Throughout the Life Cycle of a Group

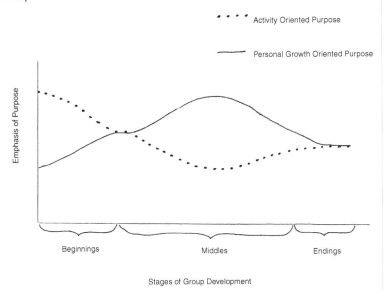

FIGURE 2. The Use of Activities in Stages of Group Development

BEGINNINGS

Characteristics of Activity:
low skill demand
includes all members at same level
    (even if varying skill levels
    exist among members)
low competitiveness
low prescriptiveness
high worker controls
high worker assistance
higher level of interactiveness
    as group proceeds through beginnings
emphasizes commonalities

Role of Activity:
helps members feel comfortable with medium
    (specific art, sport, etc.)
helps members feel accepted into the group
addresses uneasy feelings about activity
    (low minimum competence required)
allows for group norms to be set
    (acceptance of each person's
    participation, working together)
members' attitude about activity serves as
    barometer of members' comfort in group

**Relationship of Activity to
Group Purpose:**
mastery of activity emphasized
self growth purpose secondary

MIDDLES

Characteristics of Activity:
higher level of minimum competence
higher member control
    (can be chosen at members' will or
    put aside at members' will)
flexible

Role of Activity:
initiates verbal discussion
allows for more individual expression
    and emotional investment
    (individual projects of own
    or part in larger project
    such as drama or dance)
allows for risk taking
development of skills
less central in focus of verbal discussion
illustrates differences among members
    (as opposed to commonalities
    as in beginnings)

**Relationship of Activity to
Group Purpose:**
self growth purpose emphasized
mastery of activity secondary

ENDINGS

Characteristics of Activity:
return to high worker initiated control
individualized minimum competence level
deemphasizes competitive qualities
involves the whole group
explained by worker as part of termination phase

Role of Activity:
initiates feelings about termination
stimulates discussion about termination
provides stability in group
puts closure on group
expresses feelings symbolically
reminisce
unites group
more central as focus of group
    (needs to be completed in remaining sessions)
symbolizes what has been achieved in group
    (verbally and non-verbally)

**Relationship of Activity to
Group Purpose:**
the two purposes need to be discussed, linked and
    evaluated
activity needs to take precedence when remaining
    time is limited
    (the art, dance, etc., needs to be completed)

REFERENCES

Boyd, Neva, L. (1938). "Play as a Means of Social Adjustment," in *New Trends in Group Work*. New York: Association Press, pp. 210-220.

Brandler, Sondra and Roman, Camille P. (1991). *Group Work: Skills and Strategies for Effective Interventions*. New York: The Haworth Press, Inc.

Brockway, Julie Stein. (1999). *The Purposeful Use of Activities in Group Work Practice*. Lectures and Discussion, Hunter College of the City University of New York, School of Social Work.

Brown, Leonard N. (1991). *Groups for Growth and Change*. New York: Longman.

Coyle, Grace, L. (1947). "Group Work as a Method in Recreation," *The Group*, IX, April.

Delgado, Melvin. (1983). "Activities and Hispanic Groups: Issues and Suggestions," in Middleman, Ruth R., ed., *Activities and Action in Group Work*. New York: The Haworth Press. pp. 85-96.

Dromi, P.G. and Krampf, Z. (1986). "Programming Revisited: The *Miftan* Experience," *Social Work with Groups*, Vol. 9(1), Spring.

Garland, James, Jones, Hubert and Kolodny, Ralph. (1973). "A Model for Stages of Development in Social Work Groups," In Saul Bernstein, (ed.) *Explorations in Social Work*, Boston: Milford House, Inc.

Garvin, Charles D. (1997). *Contemporary Group Work*, 3rd ed., Boston: Allyn and Bacon.

Getzel, George, S. (1983). "Poetry Writing Groups and the Elderly: A Reconsideration of Art and Social Group Work," in Middleman, Ruth R., ed., *Activities and Action in Group Work*. New York: The Haworth Press. pp. 65-76.

Glassman, Urania and Kates, Len. (1990). *Group Work: A Humanistic Approach*. Newbury Park: Sage Publications.

Henry, Sue. (1992). *Group Skills in Social Work: A Four Dimensional Approach*. 2nd ed. Pacific Grove, California: Brooks/Cole Publishing Company.

Kurland, Roselle. (1978). "Planning: The Neglected Component of Group Development, *Social Work with Groups*. Vol. 1(2), pp. 173-178.

Kurland, Roselle. (1999). *Stages of Group Development: Beginning, Middle, Ending*. Unpublished handout, Hunter College of the City University of New York, School of Social Work.

Kurland, Roselle and Salmon, Robert. (1998a). "Purpose: A Misunderstood and Misused Keystone of Group Work Practice," *Social Work with Groups*. Vol. 21(3), pp. 5-17.

Kurland, Roselle and Salmon, Robert. (1998b). *Teaching a Methods Course in Social Work with Groups*. Alexandria, VA: Council on Social Work Education.

Malekoff, Andrew. (1997). *Group Work With Adolescents: Principles and Practice*. New York: The Guilford Press.

Middleman, Ruth R. (1968). *The Non-Verbal Method in Working with Groups*, New York: Association Press.

Northen, Helen. (1988). *Social Work with Groups*, 2nd ed. New York: Columbia University Press.

Ross, Andrew L. and Bernstein, Norman D. (1976). "A Framework for the Use of Group Activities," *Child Welfare*, Vol. LV(9).

Schnekenburger, E. (1995). "Waking the Heart Up: A Writing Group's Story," *Social Work with Groups*, Vol. 18(3).

Schwartz, William. (1976). "Between Client and System: The Mediating Function." In Robert W. Roberts and Helen Northen, eds. *Theories of Social Work with Groups*, pp. 171-197. New York: Columbia University Press.

Shulman, L. (1971). "Program in Group Work: Another Look," In *The Practice of Group Work*, edited by W. Schwartz and S. Zalba, pp. 221-40. New York: Columbia University Press.

Toseland, Ronald W. and Rivas, Robert F. (1998). *An Introduction to Group Work Practice*. 3rd ed. Boston: Allyn and Bacon.

Tuckman, Bruce, W. (1965). "Developmental Sequence in Small Groups." *Psychological Bulletin*, 63(6).

Vinter, Robert D. (1974). "Program Activities: An Analysis of Their Effects on Participant Behavior," in Sundel, M., Glasser, P., Sarri, R., and Vinter, R., *Individual Change Through Small Groups*. New York: The Free Press.

Wilson, Gertrude and Ryland, Gladys. (1949). *Social Group Work Practice*, Boston: Houghton-Mifflin.

Whittaker, James K. (1974). "Program Activities: Their Selection and Use in a Therapeutic Milieu," in Sundel, M., Glasser, P., and Vinter, R., *Individual Change Through Small Groups*. New York: The Free Press.

Groups-on-the-Go:
Spontaneously Formed Mutual Aid Groups
for Adolescents in Distress

Jana Jagendorf
Andrew Malekoff

SUMMARY. This paper presents groups-on-the-go, spontaneously formed groups for adolescents in distress. Groups-on-the-go is an extension of Fritz Redl's concept of life-space interviewing, which is used to address adolescents' direct, here-and-now life experiences. The two major tasks of life-space interviewing are: (1) clinical exploitation of life events and (2) emotional first aid on the spot. This article goes one step further, adding a third feature, (3) mutual aid in the moment. This article will describe and illustrate groups-on-the-go, discuss the challenges of this spontaneous approach, and offer guidelines for its effective use. *[Article copies available for a fee from The Haworth Document Delivery Service: 1-800-HAWORTH. E-mail address: <docdelivery@haworthpress.com> Website: <http://www.HaworthPress.com> © 2005 by The Haworth Press, Inc. All rights reserved.]*

Jana Jagendorf, CSW, and Andrew Malekoff, ACSW, are both with North Shore Child and Family Guidance Center, 480 Old Westbury Road, Roslyn Heights, NY. Ms. Jagendorf is a social worker in the Center's Intensive Support Program, a school based program, and Mr. Malekoff is the agency's director of program development.

This article was presented at Symposium XXI, Association for the Advancement of Social Work with Groups, Denver, Colorado, in October 1999.

This article was originally published in *Social Work with Groups*, Vol. 22 (4) © 2000 by The Haworth Press, Inc.

[Haworth co-indexing entry note]: "Groups-on-the-Go: Spontaneously Formed Mutual Aid Groups for Adolescents in Distress." Jagendorf, Jana, and Andrew Malekoff. Co-published simultaneously in *Social Work with Groups* (The Haworth Press, Inc.) Vol. 28, No. 3/4, 2005, pp. 229-246; and: *A Quarter Century of Classics (1978-2004): Capturing the Theory, Practice, and Spirit of Social Work with Groups* (ed: Andrew Malekoff, and Roselle Kurland) The Haworth Press, Inc., 2005, pp. 229-246. Single or multiple copies of this article are available for a fee from The Haworth Document Delivery Service [1-800-HAWORTH, 9:00 a.m. - 5:00 p.m. (EST). E-mail address: docdelivery@haworthpress.com].

Available online at http://www.haworthpress.com/web/SWG
doi:10.1300/J009v28n03_15

KEYWORDS. Groups, adolescents, life-space interviewing, mutual aid

This article introduces *groups-on-the-go*, spontaneously formed, school-based mutual aid groups for adolescents in distress. Groups-on-the-go is an extension of Redl's life-space interviewing (1966, 35-67), the purpose of which is to address problems in adolescents' direct, here-and-now life experience. Group workers must be problem focused, clear about goals, and active in the pursuit of their aims. However, they must also be prepared for emergent problems that occur in the life of the group, to expect the unexpected, to be ready for "group work on the go" (Malekoff, 1997, viii). This article goes one step further from addressing problems in a previously formed and functioning group, to taking on problems by spontaneously forming a new time-limited group.

The two major tasks of life-space interviewing are: (1) clinical exploitation of life events and (2) emotional first aid on the spot (Redl, 1966, 41). This article adds a third feature, (3) mutual aid in the moment by forming groups-on-the-go that can range in time from a few minutes, to a longer encounter, and can extend to a few additional follow up meetings.

Groups-on-the-go adds the peer group to the helping mix, tapping what students have to offer one another in moments of distress. A noteworthy obstacle to forming groups-on-the-go is wariness of school administrators and faculty who may fear that forming such groups will upset the routine and structure of the school day. This article will describe and illustrate groups-on-the-go, discuss the challenges of this spontaneous approach, and offer guidelines for its effective use. The setting is an alternative school for high school students identified with serious emotional disturbances. More on the setting will be described later.

ON INSTITUTIONAL CULTURE, ADVOCACY AND SOCIAL WORK WITH ADOLESCENTS

Social workers often spend their time in host settings dominated by allied professions and disciplines. One example is the public school. Social workers must be prepared to advocate for service components that may not be easily understood or accepted by allied professionals. Advocacy is not a *choice* for social workers, it is a *duty*. An unconventional approach, such as groups-on-the-go, requires advocacy and education.

The role of a social worker in a school assumes making interventions beyond individual students or circumscribed groups of students. The system itself, including all of its subsystems (teachers, pupil personnel staff, administration), can be a target of intervention. A distinction must be made between purposeful and professional advocacy and chronic griping about obstacles and challenges posed by a complex organization. As social workers struggle to contribute to even modest gains that influence the structure, culture, and tone of an institution, they become valued role models for students and faculty/staff who previously felt disempowered and hopeless regarding even the possibility of change.

GROUP WORK IN A SCHOOL: EDUCATING THE EDUCATORS

Group work in a school setting tends to generate a range of reactions. The noise, movement, and energy that are produced can lead to requests to "quiet down," puzzled looks and questions about the value of groups that depart from activity other than quiet discussion, and admonitions against laughter or any high spirited good fun not perceived as "serious business."

Good group work practice with adolescents requires a planning process that focuses on gaining sanction from school/agency administration, developing a clear purpose, selecting and screening members carefully, attending to the structural details (i.e., time and space) of the effort, and identifying appropriate content and materials for the group to meet its goals (Malekoff, 1997, 53-80; Kurland, 1978). However, in the ever changing dynamic of the "school day," spontaneous interventions are often necessary.

A critical component of this discussion is the importance of gaining administrative support for groups-on-the-go. When a number of students are unaccounted for at the same time during the school day, the reaction can range from a "here we go again" shrug of the shoulders to general alarm about their whereabouts. Group workers implementing groups-on-the-go must pay attention to administrative details, such as obtaining passes for permission to leave class. They must also be prepared to describe the value of the intervention and demystify the process for the gatekeepers in the school who might otherwise squash such efforts.

When an individual student requires an unplanned intervention to clarify a scheduling problem or address a crisis or receive guidance, school personnel more readily accept the need for a one-on-one approach to providing assistance. However, when the unplanned intervention is a spontaneous gathering of a group of students (perceived by some as a mob) eyebrows are raised, usually a preamble to an inquisition. Disapproval looms as a sense of order and control in the school building is threatened by the radical departure that such a gathering represents. Group workers must be prepared to "defend" their action and to do it in a way that is not defensive. They must assume the role of *educator* as well as advocate (more on this subject later). This is not an easy task and one that takes maturity, a systems perspective, and political acumen.

HOW GROUPS-ON-THE-GO GOT GOING

The origin of groups-on-the-go is illustrated in the author's (Jagendorf) reminiscence.

It was my worst nightmare. I was at my job for a little over two months when my colleague told me she would not be in the next day. She was attending a conference on Oppositional Defiant Disorder in Adolescents, a diagnosis that many of our clients had been given. Paula informed me that not only would she be attending the conference but the social workers and psychologists from the other units would also be at the conference. "You might need to be available to handle some of their kids too, if any crises arise." Great, no problem I thought. I can barely handle my kids and I'm supposed to be available to work with kids I don't know?

Each social worker has a case load of about 12 adolescents in this alternative school program for students who were identified as having serious emotional disturbances. One of our goals was to prevent them from being placed in institutions. The idea was for them to remain at home and in their community while attending school in the most appropriate, least restrictive setting.

How was I going to manage four other workers' students? I barely slept that night. I prayed for a blizzard so that the school would be closed. I felt ill and thought, well, maybe I am coming down with something and need to call in sick.

The next day came sans snow and I found myself with little clinical support at school. Sam was in my room for his 8:30 AM session. He was brooding and quiet, playing with a puzzle and talking about music, when someone knocked on the door. It was Cara stating that she could come to see me this period because she was "in crisis" and had a pass from her teacher. "Well, I'm with Sam at the moment. Can you come back?" She looked at me incredulously, and said, "No!" I asked Sam if he would mind going back to class and he said, "Yes!" Cara stood in the doorway, so I said, "Come in. Let me try to figure something out."

I wanted to assess the severity of the crisis so I asked her if she could say a little of what the problem was in front of Sam. She began to recount an incident she had with a boy she broke up with and her guilty feeling that she was happy seeing another boy while her previous boyfriend seemed so hurt. Sam mumbled something and Cara and I looked at him. "What did you say, Sam?" I asked. "You can't always be responsible for everyone else," he said. I asked him to say more and he proceeded to ask Cara whether she had first broken up with her boyfriend or if she had cheated on him. She said that she broke up with him and that one month later began going out with another boy. Sam seemed upset as he told Cara that it wasn't her fault and that the same thing had happened to him.

"You broke up with Meg?" she asked.

"No, she broke up with me and is going out with Sal."

Cara and Sam discussed going out with students in the school and how difficult it was to be in such a small program. You could not avoid seeing someone and everyone knows your business.

The bell rang and it was time for the next student to come in.

"Are you feeling better, Cara?" Sam asked.

"Yeah, thanks Sam," Cara replied.

Sam said, "That's okay. I was just playing with a puzzle anyway." He left for class, smiling.

A little later that morning, I was in an individual meeting with Jill when someone knocked loudly on my door and opened it. I had no idea what this student's name was, but I had seen her in the hallways. A frazzled teacher stood next to her. Jonette, a tall, heavy set and muscular looking girl dressed in hip hop style, looked angry. "Jonette will not stay in class and seems very agitated. Her counselor is out at some conference," the teacher stated sarcastically. "Can you see her?" Jonette and Jill said hello to each other and seemed pretty friendly. Jill said she could go back to class. I asked Jill, who had been talking about a school issue, if it was okay for Jonette to join us. She said, "Yeah, I don't have much to say today." I turned to Jonette and asked her how she would feel if Jill stayed in the room. "Jill's cool, that would be okay," she said. At that moment Maura, a student who worked with my colleague Paula, opened the door and pushed past Jonette, a dangerous thing to do. The hierarchy was forming in front of my eyes. Maura was dressed in gothic look, lots of chains hanging from her waist, black lipstick and lots of black eye liner. She threw the pass in my direction and snarled, "I have a pass to see you. My fucking counselor is never in when I need her." She sat down in one of the chairs and glared at me. I asked both girls if it was okay for Maura to join us and they said it was fine. Over the next thirty minutes Maura and Jonette were able to share with Jill the issues that brought them into the room and all three girls were able to support and confide in each other.

The author recalls: the rhythm of the day was laid out for me. During every session, I was interrupted by another student, either walking in or brought to me by a teacher with an issue that needed to be addressed.

ON TRAFFIC JAMS AND CAR POOLING IN THE EXPRESS LANE

In the beginning, groups-on-the-go occurred spontaneously. Although the group worker's colleagues, in the preceding illustration, were out of the building that day, the need for students to be seen still had to be met. Any attempt to meet the needs of all students who had issues to discuss on a day that staffing was so sparse created a traffic jam. The solution was like the concept of car pooling. One person in a car creates so much traffic. If you're headed in the same destination more or less, why not travel together. For the group worker the concept was not so farfetched. Group planning time was minimal. Group composition, while carefully determined, was unpredictable. Nevertheless, stating a purpose remained constant. What these impromptu gatherings offered was *mutual aid* in the face of a crisis.

GUIDELINES FOR GROUPS-ON-THE-GO

Pay Attention to Process, Structure and Boundaries

The first step is to get consent from each of the group members. Of course if a student is in the middle of a difficult or deeply personal meeting it is important to allow them to continue without interruption. Even if this is not the case it is necessary to be attuned to subtle cues suggesting uneasiness about sharing a meeting. Boundaries must be respected. A successful group-on-the-go can be helpful to students who are used to isolating themselves as they experience the benefits of sharing a meeting and offering assistance.

Composition is not haphazard in forming a group-on-the-go. As a program social worker, one is privileged to have an understanding of each potential group member's history. When working with a student/client who is blocked or hesitant about bringing an emotional issue to the surface, who can be more helpful than a peer? Kids trust kids and listen to each other when provided with a safe situation that validates their helping capacity.

Students need not feel pressured to set a time limit. If a student comes in feeling like a pressure cooker about to explode, a group-on-the-go can help them vent, offering emotional first aid on the spot to reduce the strain enough for them to go about their day without further incident. A group-on-the-go can last five minutes or an hour depending upon the need.

Emphasize Group Members' Strengths, What They Have to Offer

In group work, altruism is an empowering force. In a group-on-the-go members are asked without warning to help others and share. Because of the spontaneous nature of these groups during an unpredictable moment of crisis, a group-on-the-go can be unexpectedly intimate and powerful.

In working with adolescents, an awareness of students' strengths is crucial. For example, one student may have developed a good capacity to use insight for coping. Another might have a more advanced reasoning ability for sorting out problems. Social workers are often faced with what is equivalent to jump starting a failing battery. They may be prepared to attach the cables and spark the low battery back to life; however, another car that's running smoothly is needed to do the job. Peers meeting in a context that invites trust can provide the charge that allows a fellow student to rev his or her engine until they're up and running again. The experience can be cathartic for all who are involved in the process. Mutual aid becomes a norm and youth learn the power of being available to each other, listening and sharing.

Students who have psychiatric histories, have experienced many hospitalizations, are on medication, and have been placed in a Special Education program have often had their sense of power and health taken from them. They feel labeled by their psychiatric diagnosis and feel they are crazy, sick, and incapable of thinking clearly. Inviting a student to help a peer gives the message that the worker trusts the student's reasoning ability and thinking and that students' understanding of each other is valued. This gives the clear message that their insights, thoughts, ideas, and recommendations are believed to be worthwhile, valuable, and trustworthy.

Even a teenager without a psychiatric history might feel that the adult world looks at her or him as being incapable of thoughtful reflection and action. Yet for an adolescent who is going through a psychiatric journey, multiple hospitalizations and the need for daily medication can have a powerfully crippling effect on his or her sense of self. There is an important message in a worker's letting students know that he or she is aware of their health, resiliency, and natural courage to work through whatever brought them into treatment. There is a two-fold message that is being communicated by forming a group-on-the-go. Students discover that not only can they help themselves, but they can help others. When a student is enlisted by the worker to provide mutual aid, the message is that the worker sees strength in the student's journey rather than labeling it as a sick and crazy period of time.

Form Alliances with Relevant Others in the School

Groups-on-the-go may be seen by host administrators and faculty/staff as an excuse for students to get together and hang out, looking for ways to socialize and avoid academics. Communicating with school staff and explaining the purpose and value of such groups is a critical feature of the success of this innovative approach. Relevant others cannot be cut out of the equation or complained about or scoffed at for their lack of understanding. Group workers must be active in forming good working alliances with relevant others in the students' lives (Malekoff, 1997, 102-118).

In an in-school program, one of the challenges facing group workers in gaining administrative and faculty/staff support is that groups-on-the-go are spontaneously formed and not on the formal schedule. They can be disruptive to the day-to-day routine in school, possibly giving the impression to teachers and administrators that the workers and students are out of control. Traditional group work meetings may take place at regularly scheduled weekly or twice-weekly times. A group-on-the-go usually requires that students receive passes from teachers to be excused from class with little to no advance notice. Because constant interaction is required between the group worker and the administration and staff, it is important for the worker to communicate well with the staff in order to gain support.

Don't Disregard or Underestimate the Need for Trust, Privacy, and Confidentiality

Carelessly exposing issues that should be kept between worker and student is an obstacle to the effective use of groups-on-the-go. When a student is already involved in an individual meeting with a worker, the worker must be careful not to encourage a student to share the meeting when, in fact, he or she does not want to. Privacy must be respected. Group workers must be sure to check-in with students before allowing or encouraging an opening up of content that cannot be adequately addressed or expressed in this time-limited approach.

For example, it may be too difficult, powerful, and or embarrassing for an adolescent to deal with the intensity of a taboo issue, such as violence or alcoholism in the family, in an individual session. The worker knows which students are further along in the process of understanding and coping with these issues, and even which students have been victims of abuse. While being sensitive to confidentiality, it is important for the worker to take advantage of his or her ability to recognize appropriate commonalties when forming a group-on-the-go.

Make a Demand for Work

The social worker must be careful to guard against students trying to avoid the work that needs to be done in an individual meeting by inviting others to join in on the spot. Similarly, once a group-on-the-go is formed the members must honor the commitment reflected when they chose to participate.

The worker has to be on guard against a student's desire to hide within a group in order for his or her issue to remain unaddressed. For some students the intensity and quietness of an individual session may be exactly what is needed for an issue to surface. Another consideration is that once a group is formed the worker may be reluctant to address an issue that requires the privacy of an individual session.

Since adolescents generally want to be surrounded by peers, they usually welcome a spontaneously formed group-on-the-go. The worker must make sure that a group-on-the-go is not a social gathering or hang out period (which obviously has its place), but is an intervention providing mutual aid for students in distress. All participants are responsible for addressing the need that leads to the formation of a group-on-the-go. The group worker is responsible for keeping the group on track and focused.

Invite the Whole Person to Participate

One of the beautiful things about groups-on-the-go is that they can address crises that are not "psychiatric" in nature or related to "pathology," but that represent the normative needs of the young people. To request the help of a student in a spontaneously formed group-on-the-go is to pull the whole person in to the moment (e.g., to ask that the young man who is a drummer and resides in a group home and likes Metallica or the girl who is proud of her heritage, part Native American, part Polish, who loves to draw and hates living with her mother to join the discussion).

Since a student often does not know what to expect or why he or she is needed in a group-on-the-go, the realization alone that a fellow student is in need suggests that the "whole person" is being invited to enter the room. Adolescents who are used to a psychiatric program have lived with going from one formal group therapy experience to another. Whether it is a "Girls' Group," or "Art Therapy Group," the student is aware of the theme and the routine and may put on a therapeutic "coat" before "going to group." This unscheduled group is not on the traditional therapeutic menu. With an unannounced natural formation of a group-on-the-go, the student strolls in unprepared, unguarded, and relaxed.

Forming a group-on-the-go implies an invitation for the whole person to participate and it assumes that the worker is not the central helping person, that group members are helpers too. The following illustration brings groups-on-the-go and these vital principles of group work with adolescents to light.

JEROLD, JUANITA, AND BEV TEACH JAY HOW TO DANCE

Jay sat in session upset, dirty blonde hair over his eyes, with no expression on his face. Jay always maintained that he never smiled, not even when he was a little kid. I rarely saw him smile, and on the chance that I did, I always felt like I was witnessing something so sweet and gentle. Jay loves music and plays the keyboard. He often spoke about the music he listened to. He likes Nirvana and Korn, groups that sing about depressing, painful themes. Jay said that he was invited to Maria's sweet sixteen party this Friday and that all his friends from school were going. Jay said, "But I'm not going. And if I go, I'll stay outside and smoke cigarettes or sit in the corner like I did at the prom last year. I'll just sit like this all night." He proceeded to cross his arms, slump down in his chair and look depressed.

We talked for awhile about why Jay didn't want to go to Maria's sweet sixteen, canceling out possible options like, "Are you still in love with her?" Jay finally blurted out, "I can't dance." "No? You've never danced at a party or a concert?" I asked. "Well, I jump into the mosh pit. That's great, banging heads and pulling at people's clothes. But I don't think they'll have that at the sweet sixteen." "You're probably right Jay," I said. Then I wondered aloud, "Can you ask your little sister to teach you how to dance?" Jay was firm in his answer, "I don't want MY SISTER teaching me to dance, no way."

There was a knock on the door and Jerold bounced in. Jerold has great energy and poise. And he is a wonderful dancer. "Jerold, perfect timing. Jay, can I tell Jerold about your dilemma?" Jay seemed to shrug his response, "Sure, tell him."

"You're going to Maria's sweet sixteen, right Jerold?" I asked.

"Oh yeah," he said.

"Well, Jay doesn't want to go."

Jerold turned to Jay, "No way, how come?"

"Cause I don't know how to dance."

"You can dance, Jay," Jerold said.

"No, I don't know how. If I go I'm just going to sit in the corner or stay outside until it's over. I'll wear my torn pants and a tie-dyed shirt. Maybe they won't even let me in."

"Jerold, you're a great dancer," I said. "Do you think you could teach Jay to dance?

"Yeah, I could teach you, give you some moves. You could do it."

"What do you say, Jay? You both could come to my office, I'll lock the door and we could have a dance lesson."

I was surprised that Jay really went for the idea. I suggested adding Juanita to the lesson. She was also attending the party, and it would be good for Jay to practice dancing with a girl. Perhaps they might even dance together at the party. We arranged the best time for all of us to meet according to everyone's schedule. Jerold said he could get a tape of some good dance music from another student and we agreed to meet later on that day at 12:30. Before Jerold left I asked Jay if he wanted this to stay confidential, and he said, "No, I don't care who knows."

A little later that morning I was in a session with Bev when Juanita knocked on the door to confirm the dance session. She handed me a pass from her gym teacher, stating it was okay to miss her 12:30 class. Jay came in at that moment to check that we were still on for his dance lesson.

When both Juanita and Jay left, Bev asked me what was going on. I explained Jay's problem and Bev said that she also couldn't dance. I didn't believe that, knowing and working with Bev for about a year. But I knew she was very self conscious and uncomfortable with boys. I invited Bev to join our dance group. I told her that it made more sense in fact to have two boys and two girls and that she could watch, hang out or join in. She said she would get a pass from her teacher and would be there at 12:30.

Jay got to my room first and walked in looking apprehensive, scoping out my office to see if any of the others were there yet. "Jay, this is going to be fun. I invited Bev to join us. Is that okay?" I asked. He seemed okay with that, replying, "Yeah, that'll be good. Bev is cool."

The door swung open and Jerold entered, charged, tape in hand, smiling. Juanita walked in, looking a bit nervous. "So what are we going to do?" she asked. "We're here to help Jay by teaching him how to dance so he can have a great time this Friday at Maria's sweet sixteen party," I said. Bev opened the door and came in and I told the group I had invited

Bev too. Both Jerold and Juanita thought Bev was a good addition. I put up the 'Do Not Disturb' sign before closing and locking the door.

Juanita asked Jay about his never dancing before. He talked about the mosh pit at concerts and talked about how his father danced. He imitated his father's one and only dance move to me once and it was really funny so I asked him to show the group, thinking it would get Jay to move a bit and break the ice. He did, the group laughed and Jerold joined in and added some corny moves to Jay's.

I told the group that Jay was very athletic, aware that they didn't know that he had played football and wrestled in his other school. My guess was that he probably could dance but maybe never really tried. Jerold put the tape on and some salsa music filled the air. Juanita, who is from the Dominican Republic, yelled, "I love this music." All the kids were standing in a circle and Juanita was moving a bit to the rhythm. Jerold began to dance next to Juanita and then the two of them began to dance as we all looked on. Jay looked defeated and said, "I'll never learn to dance."

"Juanita, why don't you show Jay some steps?" I said. Juanita is now more relaxed from dancing with Jerold and begins to show Jay some moves. He starts dancing and Juanita says, "You're doing the Meringue! How do you know how to do that?" Jay says, "My mom is from Brazil, she taught me." "I knew it," said Juanita. "I knew you had Spanish blood. Oh, *then you can dance*, look, you're doing the Meringue. Salsa is even easier."

Bev began to imitate Juanita's moves and Jerold turned to her and began dancing with her. Jay concentrated and watched and danced with the others. Jerold requested I be in charge of the tape and fast forward to some other music. When a slow song came on, everyone stopped. "Did you ever dance a slow dance with a girl before?" Juanita asked Jay, laughing. Jay said no and Juanita said to hold her around the waist and to just dance. Jay looked uncomfortable and anxious.

Jerold went over to him and said, "It's mad easy, just grab her hand like this." And he grabbed Jay's hand. "Put your other hand around her back and just move." Jerold put his hand on Jay's back and there they were, Jay and Jerold slow dancing for a few seconds as we all looked on.

Then Jerold, as if catching himself in a not-so-macho-moment, broke away from Jay and turned to Juanita and said, "Or you could dance like a player, like this," and began a close and seductive dance with Juanita. She laughed and pushed him away, shouting, "Jerold!" Jerold took Juanita's hand and put his arm around her and they began to dance a waltz.

"Hey Bev, how about helping Jay with a slow dance," I said. Bev smiled and went over to Jay. They took each other's hand, Jay gently put his hand around Bev's waist and they began to dance. The bell rang and I told everyone we had to stop now. I could see how hesitant they all were to stop. "So listen, I think in order to help Jay really feel secure we need more than one dance group. What do you all think?" Jay said, "Why can't we meet again tomorrow?" I asked if everyone would like that and if it would be possible according to their class schedules. Everyone said yes and that they would talk with their teachers to get the okay.

The next day Jay came in first thing in the morning to confirm the dance group time. I was surprised to see him smiling, especially so early in the morning. At 12:30 when Jay came into my office he was dancing a combination of the Meringue and some new Salsa moves. He was bitten by the dance bug. Jerold came in, upset that he forgot to bring music and that no one seemed to have any tapes on them. He hoped that Juanita or Bev had some music on them. When the girls arrived, they said that they didn't have any music.

I showed the kids my CDs and they laughed. "Well, what's wrong with Aretha Franklin?" I asked. "You can't dance to her," said Jerold. "I mean I like her but you can't dance to Aretha," he added. I said, "Let's give it a try." Juanita laughed and said to put on the song RESPECT. I did and when the music began everyone but Jay and I started laughing. Bev, Jerold and Juanita began doing some kind of disco dance. First they all did different steps, then watching each other and dancing in a line dance perfectly mimicking each other. They were so in synch. They could have been Aretha's back-up singers, I thought to myself. As I watched them I marveled at how connected they all seemed at that moment. Bev, who was so quiet and distant and had so many issues of feeling unsafe, seemed so content and happy. They were all connected, all but Jay that is. He was again on the outside looking in.

I shouted over the music and their dancing, "Hey group, why are we here?" referring with a gesture to Jay who was not dancing but watching them in awe. "Dancing and teaching dance are two separate things. Don't forget we're here to help Jay," reminding them of the purpose of this group-on-the-go. Jerold suggested we look for a good radio station. It was difficult to get radio reception in my room without a lot of static, unless you held and moved the antenna. That was to be my role. Jerold turned the dial this way and that as Jay looked nervous and watched the clock. He found a reggae station and I grabbed the antenna.

Soon all three began dancing again and Jay looked on. Jerold stopped, walked over to Jay, and began to systematically show him a Reggae step. Slowly Jay and Jerold did the step. Bev faced Jay and began learning the dance step. She asked Jerold to slow down and asked him if he started with his left foot or right. I suggested to Jerold that as he danced he state which foot he was using.

As Jerold chanted, "Left, left, slide right," Jay kicked off his shoes and followed Jerold's steps. I watched as the smile lit Jay's face. Juanita went up to Jay, took his hands out of his pockets, and said, "Keep your hands out and move your arms like this. Move your hips too, you're too stiff." Bev demonstrated, "Like this Jay, you've got to feel the music." The music continued to play and Jerold danced next to Jay, chanting, "Left, left, slide right." Juanita and Bev danced in front of Jay, with him and guiding him along. And then magically, in the moment with the music, the group was dancing together. "He got it! He's dancin'," Bev shouted. "Yeah, Jay!" Juanita yelled. "I knew you could dance," said Jerold. Jay continued to smile.

The bell rang and students' voices filled the hallway. I dropped the antenna and static muffled sounds drowned out the Reggae music. Everyone stopped dancing. Complaints and requests like, "Come on, Jana. Can't we dance longer?" were sent my way. The door opened up and Isaac entered, ready to go with me to the guidance counselor's office.

"Well, Jay, how are you feeling about the party?" I asked. "Maybe I will dance," Jay declared. "All right!" shouted Jerold. Bev began to clap and we all joined in. The dance group spilled out of my room and I watched them all dancing together down the hallway on their way to their next class.

DISCUSSION

In this illustration the dynamics of mutual aid are apparent (Shulman, 1999, 1985/86). Discussing a taboo subject ("I can't dance."); mutual support ("You're doing the meringue, how do you know how to do that?"); mutual demand ("Don't forget, we're here to help Jay."); rehearsal ("And then magically, in the moment with the music, the group was dancing together."); sharing data ("Jerold walked over to Jay and started to systematically show him how to do a Reggae step."); and strength-in-numbers phenomenon (not going it alone) all are in evidence.

In a surprise twist, the group worker learned that when the teachers discovered that Jay was learning how to dance, rather than expressing disapproval they were excited and supportive. They knew about how sad he had been and of his history of depression and hospitalization. They recognized the benefits of this group-on-the-go with its clear purpose and activity that spilled into the hallways with an infectious spirit.

Far from coming into conflict with the culture of the school building, groups-on-the-go can positively influence the school culture. Faith in mutual aid and what students have to offer, willingness to take the risk of forming a group-on-the-go, and readiness to navigate obstacles and manage logistics can impact favorably on the school environment. By emphasizing students' strengths, maintaining an optimistic outlook that problems can be solved, and never losing sight of the normative experiences of young people who are most often identified by deficits, a group-on-the-go can go a long way to adding spirit and character to a school (or other setting inhabited by children and teens), instilling a sense of hope in both the youth and adults who inhabit such a sacred space together.

AFTERMATH:
"YOU CAN'T BE ALONE
BECAUSE YOU'RE STUCK WITH US"

When groups-on-the-go become a part of a program culture the inevitable occurs: Those on the giving end of help eventually become those on the receiving end, emphasizing the give and take that is at the heart of mutuality. The article closes with an illustration of this process.

> I heard yelling in the hallway and opened my door to see Jerold screaming, kicking the wall, and punching his fist over and over again into the door. His screams were filled with both rage and sadness and the impact of his hand hitting the metal door was sure to be painful. Jerold's feelings overwhelmed him. His fury was too great for him to handle and exploded from him both physically and verbally. Students stopped in the hallway, not moving or talking, just watching Jerold. When I called his name he looked around as if coming out of a trance. Seeing all the students staring added shame to his other painful emotions as he took off down the hallway. Running ahead were Juanita and Jay. When they caught up to him I couldn't hear what they were saying but the quiet tones of

their voices were obviously soothing to him. We all spoke a few minutes in the hallway and walked together with Jerold back to my office, Juanita and Jay on either side of him. Jay said, looking at Jerold's bruised hand, "That looks like it really hurts." Jerold cried and said, "Everything hurts." Malcolm, who had just been talking to Jerold before the outburst occurred, asked if it was something he had done. I said that everyone was here because they cared about him and asked if he could confide in his friends.

Jerold cried and words exploded from him in a rapid fire explanation of his fears of loneliness and rejection. He said, "My father left me when I was three and you, Malcolm, said you didn't want to hang out with me this weekend and laughed about it. I don't know, I just exploded. I know you all think I'm *all that* because I have a lot of stuff–computers and phat clothes and things–but I buy them so that you all want to hang out with me." Each friend then shared similar stories. Malcolm spoke of never meeting his father and thinking that if he got a driver's license and car that he would be more popular. Juanita spoke of her father's drug addiction and not having seen him in many years and feeling insecure about herself. Jay said, "I'm not doing anything this weekend. Why don't you hang with me?" Malcolm said, "I was just joking. I didn't know you'd take it so seriously. Now I know to be more careful about things like this." Jerold said, "I just need people around me a lot. That's my problem. I don't like being alone." Juanita gave him a hug and said, "You can't be alone because you're stuck with us."

CONCLUSION

On just about every corner in America throughout the generations from Woodstock '69 to Woodstock '99, from soda fountains to Starbucks, one can see teens hanging out with each other. When else is the need to feel a sense of belonging in a group more powerful than during the adolescent years? This is the era when cognitive complexity, self reflection, and deeper levels of understanding are developing. Adolescence is also a time of contradictions, when wanting to be left alone and among others are equally compelling needs. What makes groups-on-the-go *go* is that adolescents, during this unbridled and spirited time of life, are best equipped to help each other. Who better than a fellow teen to acknowledge the dignity of all adolescents, whether one has a psychiatric history or is stumbling along attempting to find a little grace while figuring out new found personal territory in the search for identity. Amid all of this, the ability of adolescents to support one another is the true gift of groups-on-the-go.

REFERENCES

Kurland, R. (1978). Planning–The Neglected Component of Group Development. *Social Work with Groups*, 1(2), 173-178.

Malekoff, A. (1997). Planning in Group Work: Where We Begin. *Group Work with Adolescents: Principles and Practice*. New York: The Guilford Press, 53-80.

Malekoff, A. (1997). What's Going On In There?: Alliance Formation with Parents Whose Adolescent Children Join Groups. *Group Work with Adolescents: Principles and Practice*. New York: The Guilford Press, 102-118.

Redl, F. (1966). Life-Space Interview–Strategy and Techniques. In F. Redl (Ed.) *When We Deal with Children: Selected Readings*. New York: The Free Press, 35-67.

Shulman, L. (1999). The Skills of Helping Individuals, Families, Groups and Communities (Fourth Edition). Itasca, Illinois: F.E. Peacock, 303-312.

Shulman, L. (1985/86). The Dynamics of Mutual Aid. In A. Gitterman and L. Shulman (Eds.) Group Practice as Shared Interaction [Special Issue]. *Social Work with Groups*, 8(4).

White Gloves and Cracked Vases:
How Metaphors Help Group Workers
Construct New Perspectives and Responses

Trudy K. Duffy

SUMMARY. The metaphor is one of the most basic mechanisms for understanding our experiences. When we construct metaphors, we use both sides of the brain, the intuitive and rational, with the potential of generating new understanding, new realities, and new behaviors. This article promotes the creation of metaphors as a way for group workers to reflect on their practice. An image of a group offers different dimensions for consideration than verbal descriptions. Metaphor-making and elaboration can be used for learning in the classroom, supervision and practice. *[Article copies available for a fee from The Haworth Document Delivery Service: 1-800-HAWORTH. E-mail address: <docdelivery@haworthpress.com> Website: <http://www.HaworthPress.com> © 2005 by The Haworth Press, Inc. All rights reserved.]*

Trudy K. Duffy, MSW, is Clinical Professor, Boston University School of Social Work.

The author wishes to thank students, clinicians, and colleagues–Lois Levinsky, Christine Saulnier, Linda Schiller and Jim Garland–for their examples and inspiration for this article.

This article was originally published in *Social Work with Groups*, Vol. 24 (3/4) © 2001 by The Haworth Press, Inc.

[Haworth co-indexing entry note]: "White Gloves and Cracked Vases: How Metaphors Help Group Workers Construct New Perspectives and Responses." Duffy, Trudy K. Co-published simultaneously in *Social Work with Groups* (The Haworth Press, Inc.) Vol. 28, No. 3/4, 2005, pp. 247-257; and: *A Quarter Century of Classics (1978-2004): Capturing the Theory, Practice, and Spirit of Social Work with Groups* (ed: Andrew Malekoff, and Roselle Kurland) The Haworth Press, Inc., 2005, pp. 247-257. Single or multiple copies of this article are available for a fee from The Haworth Document Delivery Service [1-800-HAWORTH, 9:00 a.m. - 5:00 p.m. (EST). E-mail address: docdelivery@haworthpress.com].

doi:10.1300/J009v28n03_16

KEYWORDS. Metaphors, group work, group therapy, social work education

Metaphors are said to structure how we perceive, how we think, and what we do. When group workers create images or metaphors of their groups, they have access to the structures they are using–their viewpoints and inferences. They can move beyond jargon and fixed interpretations to new realities, understanding, and self-awareness. Metaphor-making is simple, but it can add dimension to group workers' reflective processes–drawing upon both sides of the brain, or "imaginative rationality" (Lakof and Johnson, 1980). The purpose of the article is to illustrate how metaphors can enlighten group work practice. The author includes a definition of metaphor, a brief review of the literature, illustrations of how to create and carefully use metaphors, and examples of metaphors as means for integrating theory and method, developing self-awareness, reinforcing skills, and tracking progress.

DEFINITION

Lakoff and Johnson (1980) state that the "essence of metaphor is experiencing one kind of thing in terms of another" (p. 5). The word metaphor is derived from the Greek *meta*, meaning above or over and *phorein*, meaning to carry from one place to another. The root words imply that the image created is more than a simple substitution for what is already known. Richards (1936) stated that meaning emerges from the interaction of the total metaphor–the thing signified and the image–allowing those involved to conceptualize data in a different way and generate new ideas. It is the "semantic impertinence" (Richards, 1936) or the "essential doubleness" of metaphors (Burke, 1935:1965) that gives us perspective.

Olds (1992) said:

> Metaphors are 'meaning transports' which extend our level of understanding by comparison, or some might argue by smuggling extra dimensions into our analysis. In either case they enrich the field of potential comprehension. (p. 24)

LITERATURE REVIEW

The clinical literature reflects an interest in the use of metaphors, often as integral to therapeutic work, but also as a primary method (metaphor therapy) (Barker, 1996; Cirillo and Crider, 1995; Erickson and Rossi, 1980; Gergen, 1990; Kopp, 1995). Group work literature illustrates multiple uses of metaphors in the group process (Camblin, Stone, and Merritt, 1990; Gans, 1991; Gatz and Christie, 1991; Katz, 1983; McClure, 1989; Sunderland, 1997-98). Several authors used metaphors from the group's talk to conceptualize and track group development (Christiansen, 1990; Srivastva and Barrett, 1988). Barrett and others utilized the concept of generative metaphors for large group and organizational changes (Barrett and Cooperrider, 1990; Barrett, Thomas, and Hocevar, 1995). Middleman and Wood (1985, 1993) promoted visual, imaginative methods of teaching and practice. Larsen-McKay (2000) and Bernstein (1998) studied the use of metaphors in teaching and training. This article differs in that it accents the *worker's* metaphor of the group as a way of learning. The following is a detailed example of this use of metaphor in a classroom.[1]

DRAWING TOGETHER METHOD AND THEORY

As a warm-up for group work class, the teacher rolled out a sheet of mural paper and asked the students (one at a time) to draw a picture of something they had feelings about, related to their practice. One student drew a pair of white gloves with little buttons at the wrists. She explained that this was how she saw her women's group–the members were so nice and so supportive, but little work was getting done. She found that she did not want to go to group meetings. She offered that she came from a family that dealt openly with differences, so she was accustomed to frankness and contest.

Among the images drawn, the white gloves attracted the most interest and the class chose to focus on them.[2] The teacher then worked with the class to make associations, to explore the meaning of the image in relation to the group that it signified, to consider relevant theory, and to develop practice alternatives.

Students quickly offered associations: "being proper," "nice," "polite," "keeping clean," "the white gloves test," "society," "church," and "protection." The student/worker clarified that the group was for women who had been sexually and physically abused. The associations took on greater meaning. The women presented well, but may not have felt particularly clean, nice, or safe. "Taking off the gloves," in boxing terms, meant no fight, but it also meant that participants would have to somehow face their differences, perhaps get "down and dirty." Asked how the women felt about the pace of the group, the worker identified one member who seemed quite satisfied with the way things were and one member who seemed impatient (like the worker, herself). The class began to see the two group members as dealing with the same issue (the development of trust, the risk of alienation), but being on different ends of the continuum.

The teacher drew in available theory, asking them to consider the effects of trauma (Herman, 1992; Van der Kolk and Fisler, 1995) and the importance of establishing safety and self-soothing skills in the beginning of the group (Schiller and Zimmer, 1994). She asked them to consider Schiller's model of group development (1995, 1997), which highlights the importance, for women, of building a relational base and establishing a felt sense of safety before challenging each other. This model contrasts with traditional group stage models (Garland, Jones, and Kolodny, 1965; Northen, 1969; Shulman, 1999; Tuckman, 1965) that place primary power struggles in the early stages of the group. Conflict in women's groups, according to Schiller (1995, 1997), occurs within the context of connections, initial differentiation, mutuality and interpersonal empathy.[3]

The class worked back and forth between the image, the group, the worker, and theory, being careful to stay with the worker in constructing meaning. The white glove metaphor made known the tension the worker was experiencing at that particular point in the group's life and offered some clues about the source of that tension. The metaphor helped everyone appreciate the vulnerability of the women in this group and to think of their cautiousness in a more complex way.

The discussion turned to possible approaches. In metaphoric terms, the members could experiment with the gloves–take them off one at a time, take both off briefly at first, and put them back on when things got scary; the worker could experiment with some kid gloves–try approaching the women's fears more gently. In concrete terms, the worker could: (1) take time to assess with the members how they felt the group was going and what they were ready to do at this point–did they feel safe enough to go deeper into their experiences of abuse? (2) affirm the steps they had already taken to make connections with each other and to assure safety, (3) acknowledge and support the expression of differences, and (4) share the worker's own tension about the pace and reach for any ambivalence or difference in viewpoints. To do the latter, the worker might consider using the white glove metaphor directly to see if it had any meaning for the members. This should be offered carefully, however, and with a willingness to accept the members' interpretations without judgement.

In the example above, consideration of the metaphor, in conjunction with practice theory, helped the worker develop greater empathy for the group members; she approached the next session with more energy and direction. In addition, because of its collective work and shared meaning around the metaphor, the class as-a-whole moved to a new level of cohesion. "There is a unique way in which the maker and the appreciator[s] of a metaphor are drawn closer to one another" (Cohen, 1970, p. 6).

METAPHOR-MAKING AND REFLECTION

Because the human conceptual system is metaphoric in nature (Lakoff and Johnson, 1980), the creation of metaphors comes easily. Here are some spontaneous responses given by group workers, when asked the question, "What image or metaphor comes to mind when you think of your group?"

- a bowl of chili that has different levels of spiciness on different days (but you're not always in the mood for chili)
- a couch that is comfortable but has a few broken springs
- a warm nest lined with soft feathers (for women rape victims until they are ready to fly)
- a hard workout that hurts, but is good for you (men's group)
- the very end of the toothpaste and you squeeze out everything that you can. You wonder, "Will you get anything?" "Will it glop out?"
- the New York stock exchange
- a rock tumbler (smoothing rough edges, bringing out color and shine)
- A mine field (the old staff knew where the explosives were, but the new staff did not know)
- Vases that have cracks in them–parents who have lost custody of their children because of addiction and other problems. The vases come in all shapes, sizes and colors; some are more damaged than others, requiring different time periods for restoration. The leader and the group are the glue helping to mend the cracks, so that eventually the vases can hold water and flowers (the children).

Construction and exploration of metaphors, as a reflective process, can be done in the context of a class, supervision, or consultation group. This has the advantage of multiple perspectives.[4] Metaphoric reflection can also be done individually. It is particularly useful when a worker is feeling stuck or is puzzled about something that is happening (or not happening) in the group.

DEVELOPING SELF-AWARENESS

Metaphors allow group workers to explore their feelings about their group. The worker who described the bowl of chili, representing a teen-age boys' group at a court clinic, said that he could not predict whether the chili would be spicy or not and whether he would be in the mood for such a dish. A number of questions come to mind, still staying with the metaphor. For example: Did the worker, coming from a different culture, race, ethnicity, and class, have different "tastes" than the members? Was he unfamiliar and uncomfortable with the spiciness of the slang, swears, and posturing of the members? How did he understand their behavior? What were his competencies in cooking? Could he rely on the cooking skills of the members? What did he know about the in-gredients–the steps, amounts, and methods of cooking that would result in a melding but differentiation of flavors? Did he know when to stir the pot? Was there a possibility that the chili could get too hot and, if so, what could he do to prevent this? For example, had he developed clear group norms and structures and had he ensured that the institution had a safety plan, if he needed backup? Sometimes dilemmas can be solved through the metaphor itself, without clarification and interpretation. The point is that if workers have greater self-awareness and understand the dimensions of their groups more fully, then they can move to a dif-ferent stance or action plan.

Sometimes metaphors can be introduced by a supervisor or colleague to generate new meaning. For example, a practitioner who led a group of school-aged, very active boys told her supervisor how exhausted and discouraged she was about her experience. She explained that she baked cookies and brought several activities for the boys each week in order to meet their individual choices. No matter what she did, the boys were still dissatisfied and ran all over the place. The supervisor noted that there was a parallel "running around" in the worker's efforts to fill them up and make them all happy; she said spontaneously, "It's not a birthday party, you know." After a few seconds of thought, the worker was able to talk about the purpose of the group and consider that the boys' indi-vidual needs could be met, eventually, by their developing ties and learning group-based skills–expressing, listening, waiting, deciding, playing, disagreeing. She did not have to personally satisfy each member. She accepted that a number of struggles were ahead, but she left with a clearer understanding of the group and her role in its process.

REINFORCING SKILLS

Metaphors can enlighten workers about the nature of a particular kind of group and help them gain appreciation for the skills that they already have. For example, a clinician offered the metaphor of a loaf of bread for her group in a day treatment center. The group was on-going, with open membership. As the baker, she had to be flexible, working with the ingredients on hand, the "feel" of the dough, and the conditions of the environment. She said that sometimes the bread needed more flour or water; sometimes she had to knead it and other times simply let it rise in a warm place. Metaphorically, she elaborated the competence necessary for leading these often undervalued day treatment groups. She also provided a compelling image for explaining these groups to others.

TRACKING PROGRESS VIA METAPHOR SHIFTS

A metaphor of a group will often shift over time, in line with shifts in experiences and relationships. For example, a student was assigned a collection of women in a nursing home, because they were "narcissistic, whining, and demanding." Her initial metaphor for this group–elderly women looking at themselves in separate mirrors–followed the staff's descriptions. Asked how she would like to see the women at the end of the group, she said they would be looking in the mirror and seeing other women reflected there, that is, other group members. In the student's final paper, she used an entirely different metaphor. She described the group as rare animals whose environment could not sustain their needs and freedom, so they had to be brought into a closed space for protection and survival. Her basic assumptions had changed. She no longer saw the source of the problem in the individuals; rather, they were unique, vulnerable, and beautiful. She recognized the problems in the system. Her work included, therefore, attention both to the women and to the nursing home procedures and attitudes that affected them.

Passick and White (1991) asked trainees in a substance abuse counseling course to capture the essence of the therapist-client relationship.

The first metaphors invented, for example, "General Patton," often reflected the trainees' own strict attitudes toward addiction and the level of control they believed was necessary for successful treatment. At the end of the training, they invented metaphors that captured a more collaborative, appropriately responsible stance, for example, a cab driver taking passengers around an unfamiliar city, pointing out choices.

CAUTIONS

Some cautions apply to the use of metaphors. They are time-bound and context specific. They vary from culture to culture. A "full plate," for example, has very different meanings for people with and without economic advantages. People who speak different languages may come to different metaphors and hence different realities. Dichos are examples of metaphors particular to Latino clients (Zuniga, 1992). Metaphors can limit and restrict our way of thinking because they emphasize some aspect of a situation at the expense of other, perhaps equally important ones. Practitioners can sometimes be "prisoners of their metaphors," if they are unable to step back from them to see alternative realities (Rosenblatt, 1994). Discussions of metaphors can take a competitive turn and/or ignore the interpretations that make sense to the creator. Reflections should be mutually respectful and helpful, as well as fun.

Used prudently, metaphors can help us to: (1) discover dimensions of reality or meaning not previously considered; (2) operate on several, even contradictory levels, with multiple responses; (3) by-pass resistant postures; (4) create a verbal play space; (5) highlight the moment; (6) promote interaction around a shared image; (7) allow explorations that are culturally meaningful; (8) link the imaginative and the cognitive; and (9) create, sustain and transform basic assumptions about systems (Gans, 1991).

Lakoff and Johnson (1980) argued that metaphors are not simply poetic or rhetorical embellishments, but are essential to human understanding. Lordan (1996) said that social work education requires a framework that allows students to develop in a holistic way, including scientific and artistic thinking. She said simply that the whole mind must be awakened (p. 63). This article has illustrated how reflective use of metaphors can awaken the mind, how images can help group workers unpack situations that are puzzling, help integrate method and theory, reinforce skills, and develop greater self-awareness.

NOTES

1. Some details of the examples have been altered for this article.

2. The teacher asked the students to place a hand on the image that had the most meaning for them. The image with the most hands, the white gloves, by sociometric choice (Moreno), represented the central concern of the class. Before preceding with the majority choice, however, the teacher acknowledged the students in the minority and asked them to say, very briefly to the "artists" of the images they chose, what their connection was. This provided some closure for those students and moved the whole class to a single focus.

3. Schiller noted that the cutting edge of growth for many men is making close connections, but the cutting edge for many women is the ability to hold power comfortably and to engage in conflict.

4. This appears similar to dream work, often done in groups, but in this case the images are consciously created. Participants offer associations and raise questions, but the ultimate meaning is left to the metaphor-maker.

REFERENCES

Barker, P. (1996). *Psychotherapeutic metaphors.* New York: Brunner/Mazel.

Barrett, F. and Cooperrider, D. (1990). Generative metaphor intervention: A new approach for working with systems divided by conflict and caught in defensive perception. *Journal of Applied Behavioral Science,* 26(2), 219-239.

Barrett, F., Thomas, G., and Hocevar, S. (1995). The central role of discourse in large-scale change: A social construction perspective. *Journal of Applied Behavioral Science,* 31(3), 352-372.

Bernstein, J. (1998). Development of the here-and-now in training groups for prospective group counselors. Unpublished doctoral dissertation, Southern Illinois University, Carbondale, IL.

Burke, K. (1935/1965). *Permanency and change: An anatomy of purpose* (2nd rev. ed.). New York: New Republic.

Camblin, L., Stone, W., and Merritt, L. (1990). An adaptive approach to group therapy for the chronic patient. *Social Work with Groups,* 13(1), 53-65.

Christiansen, D. (1990). The use and effects of metaphors on group stage development. Unpublished doctoral dissertation, University of Northern Colorado, Greeley, CO.

Cirillo, L. and Crider, C. (1995). Distinctive therapeutic uses of metaphor. *Psychotherapy,* 32(4), 511-519.

Cohen, T. (1978). Metaphor and the cultivation of intimacy. In S. Sacks (Ed.), *On metaphor* (pp. 1-28). Chicago: University of Chicago Press.

Erickson, M. and Rossi, E. (1980). Two level communication and the micro-dynamics of trance and suggestion. In E. L. Rossi (Ed.), *The collected papers of Milton H. Erickson on hypnosis.* New York: Irvington.

Gans, J. (1991). The leader's use of metaphor in group psychotherapy. *International Journal of Group Psychotherapy,* 41(2), 127-141.

Garland, J., Jones, H., and Kolodny, R. (1965). A model for the stages of group development. In S. Bernstein (Ed.), *Explorations in group work.* Boston, MA: Boston University.

Gatz, Y. and Christie, L. (1991). Marital group metaphors: Significance in the life stages of group development. *Contemporary Family Therapy: An International Journal*, 13(2), 103-126.

Gergen, K. (1990). Metaphor, metatheory, and the social world. In D. Leary (Ed.), *Metaphors in the history of psychology* (pp. 166-185). Cambridge, MA: Cambridge University Press.

Herman, J. (1992). *Trauma and recovery*. New York: Basic Books.

Katz, G. (1983). The non-interpretation of metaphors in psychiatric hospital groups. *International Journal of Group Psychotherapy*, 33, 53-67.

Kopp, R. (1995). *Metaphor therapy*. New York: Brunner/Mazel.

Lakoff, G. and Johnson, M. (1980). *Metaphors we live by*. Illinois: University of Chicago Press.

Larsen-McKay, C. (1999). Metaphor as a teaching tool. Unpublished doctoral dissertation, Claremont Graduate University, Claremont, CA.

Lordan, N. (1996). The use of sculpt in social groupwork education. *Groupwork*, 9(1), 62-79.

McClure, B. (1989). What's a group meta-phor? *Journal for Specialists in Group Work*, 14(4), 239-242.

Middleman, R. and Wood, G. (1985). Maybe it's a priest or a lady with a hat with a tree on it, or is it a bumble bee?! Teaching group workers to see. *Social Work with Groups*, 8(1), 3-15.

Middleman, R. and Wood, G. (1993). So much for the bell curve: Constructivism, power/conflict and the structural approach to direct practice in social work. *Journal of Teaching in Social Work*, 8(1/2), 129-145.

Northen, H. (1969). *Social work with groups*. New York: Columbia University.

Olds, L. (1992). *Metaphors of interrelatedness*. New York: State University of New York Press.

Passick, P. and White, C. (1991). Challenging General Patton: A feminist stance in substance abuse treatment and training. In C. Bepko (Ed.), *Feminism and addiction*. New York: The Haworth Press, Inc.

Richards, I. (1936). *The philosophy of rhetoric*. London: Oxford University Press.

Rosenblatt, P. (1994). *Metaphors of family systems theory: Toward new constructions*. New York: Guilford.

Schiller, L. (1995). Stages of group development in women's groups: A relational model. In R. Kurland and R. Salmon (Eds.), *Group work in a troubled society*. Birmingham, NY: The Haworth Press, Inc.

Schiller, L. (1997). Rethinking stages of development in women's groups: Implications for practice. *Social Work with Groups*, 20(3), 3-19.

Schiller, L. and Zimmer, B. (1994). Sharing the secrets: The power of women's groups for sexual abuse survivors. In A. Gitterman & L. Shulman (Eds.), *Mutual aid groups, vulnerable populations, and the life cycle* (2nd ed., pp. 215-238). Itasca, IL: Peacock Publishers.

Shulman, L. (1999). *The skills of helping individuals, families, and groups* (4th ed.). New York: Columbia University Press.

Srivastva, S. and Barrett, F. (1988). The transforming nature of metaphors in group development: A study in group theory. *Human Relations*, 41(1), 31-63.

Sunderland, C. (1997-98). Brief group therapy and the use of metaphor. *Groupwork*, 10(2), 126-141.

Tuckman, B. (1965). Developmental sequence in small groups. *Psychological Bulletin*, 63, 384-399.

Van der Kolk, B. and Fisler, R. (1995). Dissociation and the fragmentary nature of traumatic memories. Overview and exploratory study. *Journal of Traumatic Stress*, 8(3), 505-525.

Zuniga, M. (1992). Using metaphors in therapy: Dichos and Latino clients. *Social Work*, 37(1), 55-60.

Will the Real Healer Please Take a Bow

Rachel Miller

The program I work in at Hillside Hospital in Glen Oaks, New York is a National Institute of Mental Health research project designed to learn more about the early years of schizophrenia. Although my work is centered in the research division of a large psychiatric hospital, the clinical care I am involved with requires me to work with patients in a continuum of care. This begins with admission and moves through inpatient to day hospital and finally outpatient departments. This means I get to know patients at their most vulnerable, when they come into the hospital for the first time, and continue to work with them as the healing process continues into the community. The groups I facilitate include a day hospital symptom management group which meets five times a week, five outpatient groups which meet once a week each, and a twice monthly family group.

It was about the third year of leading special groups for young people with schizophrenia that I learned to let go of some of the rules of group therapy in order to tap into the strengths of my clients. Maybe I needed the rules to provide me with a sense of control when I was working with an illness that by its nature means a loss of control. Possibly I needed to be fully comfortable with schizophrenia and its many mysteries before I could begin editing the rulebook, but when I started questioning I started at the top.

This article was originally published in *Social Work with Groups*, Vol. 25 (1/2) © 2002 by The Haworth Press, Inc.

[Haworth co-indexing entry note]: "Will the Real Healer Please Take a Bow." Miller, Rachel. Co-published simultaneously in *Social Work with Groups* (The Haworth Press, Inc.) Vol. 28, No. 3/4, 2005, pp. 259-266; and: *A Quarter Century of Classics (1978-2004): Capturing the Theory, Practice, and Spirit of Social Work with Groups* (ed: Andrew Malekoff, and Roselle Kurland) The Haworth Press, Inc., 2005, pp. 259-266. Single or multiple copies of this article are available for a fee from The Haworth Document Delivery Service [1-800-HAWORTH, 9:00 a.m. - 5:00 p.m. (EST). E-mail address: docdelivery@haworthpress.com].

Available online at http://www.haworthpress.com/web/SWG
doi:10.1300/J009v28n03_17

Over the first two years working in the research study, I often thought of Freud's statement that people with schizophrenia are narcissistic. I was on the watch for that narcissism but did not see it the way I had with my previous clients with personality disorder. In fact, what I did see quite frequently was a quiet kind of support and caring these so seriously ill patients were able to give each other. Over time I began to wonder if it was the illness that was narcissistic, not the person. What I mean by this is that when people have any life threatening illness, they need all their resources to take care of themselves. Thus, people hearing voices and filled with fear due to delusions or confusion retreat into themselves and have great difficulty connecting to others. This is not a narcissistic personality, but a result of and reaction to a severe illness. Once I was clear on this, I was able to begin to draw upon the real personalities of my group members.

Though many of the young people I treat have good recoveries, the events of the day that clarified my perspective involved two young people who were still experiencing serious symptoms. Pete was a tall black young man who had stopped his medication and was rehospitalized with delusions, hallucinations and manic symptoms. He had been in the hospital for six weeks when the doctor reluctantly allowed me to take him out for a grounds walk. Honestly, I was worried because he had been so violent a few weeks earlier. At that time ten health care workers had to restrain him, but he desperately needed to get out now. He contracted not to run away, and I trusted him to keep his word as he had always done so in the past. He was so down, so very sad at having a relapse when he had been absolutely certain he would be strong enough to conquer this illness without medication.

As we walked around the campus of the hospital we talked. It was a cool winter day so we did not run into many other people, patients or staff. But as we walked past the tall glass windows of the day hospital, someone began waving excitedly. Then she burst out the front doors. It was Simone, a young woman whose symptoms, delusions about a man in a store who talked to her continuously, never responded to treatment, not to Prolixin, Risperdal, Olanzapine, Clozapine, or electro convulsive therapy. She went directly to Pete, saying, "Oh Pete, it's so good to see you." Her hug was as sincere as her words. He seemed to grow taller as his sadness was transformed into joy. They were friends from group, in their own way real friends, and her words and gestures told him how important he was to her. The tears each of us cried at that moment were of love. There was no narcissism in the air that cool day.

From that day on, I knew that the group was to be a safe place, a place of empathy and connections. Forget the books and lectures. Rethink Yalom. There were stages of group development my patients would never reach and that was just fine. These young people needed one place where they could talk about what it means to be diagnosed with schizophrenia, where they could learn about their illness, where they could question their treatment and where they could openly discuss their recent terrifying symptoms. After all, how many people can really understand what it means to say, "I used to think my mother wanted to poison me." For still other patients, the group would be the only place they could relearn how to make eye contact, small talk, or simple human connections.

To create such a group atmosphere required staying focused on the group members' strengths. Some clinicians might say such severely ill patients have few strengths, that they are the least functional with the lowest level of ego functioning. Yet I had experienced so many moments of strength by group members. Stop for a moment and imagine the courage it takes to accept and deal with an illness so stigmatizing and "hopeless." They somehow found the strength to do this, especially together as a group. They had the ability to share their own harrowing experiences with those more recently ill patients. Then there was the group's strength in confronting members' noncompliance or use of substances. The capacity to project hope to new members and take it back into themselves in the process went against all my expectations. And the empathy they could demonstrate with one another often brought me to wonder at the ability of humans to care and love, even in the worst circumstances. With their strength mine also grew. I became increasingly able to experiment and explore new means to guide them. My own hopefulness for them grew.

Slowly I began to break more rules. First, I noticed that patients who had the opportunity to experience group treatment appeared to drop out of treatment less frequently (Miller and Mason, 2001). This led to my changing the treatment strategy so that patients began joining the already scheduled day hospital group sessions while still inpatient. In this way, we guaranteed that patients would have some group experience no matter what the treatment disposition following discharge. Anyone who works in a large hospital knows this meant fighting the system; after all the inpatient, day hospital and outpatient clinic were uniquely separate divisions with little interface. At first I needed permission, but now, two years later, the group has become part of the system. In fact, the inpatient staff's perception of it is so good we might get complaints if we tried to end it.

From the first, I watched to see what worked to make the group a useful experience for the patients. It appeared that anything that made them feel connected helped them feel more hopeful. However, the severity of illness made the usual interaction extraordinarily difficult for many patients. Group activities seemed to help and one by one became part of the group culture. Today, the day hospital/inpatient group begins each morning with a wake-up game of beach ball in which the group works together to keep the ball aloft. The same group ends with a round of stretches followed by three deep breaths. The concept for going around the group with stretches originated with a patient who led us in a round robin of dancing at our second annual Halloween party. The patients also have a ritual round of checking for medication compliance, a "symptom check," and a substance abuse check when needed. This not only encourages their individual and group responsibilities but helps them practice their communication skills.

There are many opportunities for group activities that tap the patients' humanity. It's silly, they laugh, but so enjoy when the group sings happy birthday with a doughnut or Junior Mint with a candle atop. When someone moves from inpatient to day hospital or outpatient, it is marked by "For S/he is a Jolly Good Fellow." Special occasions may merit a pizza party, music and a round of dancing in follow-the-leader format. Making a shower for a soon to be new mother (the doctor) or for a group member's wedding or new apartment usually requires more guidance, but normalizes and fosters pride. Every occasion is an opportunity to be seized and used.

More and more, we tapped the strengths of individual patients. Some patients sang beautifully, danced or drew. Group artists led us to explore mood through color and drawing. They filled the walls of our room with pictures and decoration. Dancers guided us to make our parties great fun. Singers and musicians made Friday's end of week groups so special that we went from awful attendance to near perfect attendance. One member's poetry hangs on the group room wall to continue to help new patients to discuss the trauma of their first hospitalization.

Perhaps the greatest feat for thirty-five of our patients was when they came together to work on a book for other patients, *So They Say I Have Schizophrenia* (Miller and Mason, in press). The group gave of themselves in the hopes of helping other people like themselves. They worked in small groups to brainstorm the book's focus and the elements to be included. Many patients came in on their own time, again and again, to proofread, edit, write chapter introductions, and draw illustrations. It took great courage to expose themselves as they revealed their stories of illness, hospitalization and their difficulties coming to grips with a diagnosis of schizophrenia. They were smart, honest and courageous. I truly believe they could only do this because of their trust in each other's support.

Each year we try new experiments. Now patients are welcome to drop in to visit their old groups simply to say hello. Healthier patients come in to advise and share their firsthand experience of getting well. Patients move almost seamlessly from group to group as their schedules require so that they can move into jobs and school; they are able to plan around health instead of around illness. Patients who were not prepared to leave the daily day hospital symptom management group could stay with that group even when they left the day program for once a week outpatient care. Bit by bit, the groups became one larger community of peers. If they did not know each other well, they knew of each other. We began to make holiday or goodbye parties to include all patients instead of individual groups *and they came.*

Like a healthy family, they (and I) learned to be flexible and creative in order to nurture each other. We had groups of two and groups of twelve. Some patients attended the group each week, some two groups a week, and others once a month. The once a month patients (due to distance or scheduling) did not drop out, and the every week patients did not get angry. They were working together, rooting for each other, spurred on by each other's accomplishments, and supportive in times of failure. When a peer was hospitalized, they visited. Some patients had remarkable recoveries while others struggled. But they did not do it alone.

When I look back to the beginning of my work with my first episode patients, I recognize the importance of using each patient's individual talents, but the real strength, the one that makes the group special, is the ability of members to care for one another. Now I see this so clearly; but in the beginning my focus was on solving each one's unique problems while somehow building cohesion. The problems were overwhelming at times, but staying focused on the cohesion appears to be the key to what I was able to learn later about empathy and caring among first episode clients. I recall clearly my very first group of first episode patients. We had been working together for many months when the hospital made a new–and short-lived–rule requiring patients to be seen in group only. One of the group member's parents had died in Egypt, and the patient, unable to return to mourn with her family, was becoming depressed. At the end of our discussion, the group decided that the patient needed to be seen individually and directed me to "tell the boss that this was absolutely necessary." There was no envy, no malice, no scape-goating or monopolizing, just simple caring from fragile young people willing to risk using their recently practiced assertiveness skills. And I did go to my boss, and I did see her individually, and she did not have a psychotic relapse.

This ability to tap into the patients' capacity to care for one another became the main focus of my role as group leader. I learned to trust the patients to confront each other when necessary and be kind to one another regularly. My mantra became, "Group communication and cohesion is the most valuable outcome of group. Everything else will follow. Only with this connection to each other can they stay honest about their illness, less fearful to face the future and able to stay in treatment."

Two weeks before writing this, I brought a young man about to move from inpatient to the day program into a nighttime outpatient group, one I hoped he would eventually join. This was very unusual because the group he was meeting was high functioning with many members working or attending school. But I knew he needed what only they could offer: hope. I did not need to prepare the group. They, too, knew what he needed. The group had been there for them when they needed it, and they were now happy to be the healers. The group members welcomed him openly; they noticed but understood his occasional distraction; and they encouraged him to believe he could recover. When he told them he was an inpatient, that he had been hearing voices and experiencing paranoia, they smiled and told him about their own hospitalizations, delusions and hallucinations. Several weeks later, as he prepared to move into outpatient, he told his day hospital group that meeting the patients in the outpatient group, who had been in his situation before and who looked normal and had normal lives now, had meant so very much to him. He said he was ready to move into that group. He was looking forward to being part of the group that had given him hope. One day not far from now he will be the one helping the next new patient, of that I am certain.

Our groups have their share of difficult patients. There are patients who fight treatment. They discontinue their medication and use substances. They might have poor insight because of the illness or have very strong defenses, usually denial. There are patients with severe difficulties with interpersonal relationships, patients who are inappropriate, hypersexual, irritable, monopolizing, grandiose, angry, or who have a variety of other problematic personality traits. At this very time there is a young man who is sexually inappropriate, with no insight, using alcohol and telling us he will do whatever he wants whenever he wants to. He attends the day hospital program, where he comes daily to our group without complaint but only participates in other groups when threatened with expulsion from the program. Some days it is hard on the group members, yet they understand he is influenced by continuing symptoms, and therefore are patient with him. I expect one day he will be able to support others as he is now supported. For the time being, the group is providing him with support to stay in treatment. Sometimes that is all we can hope for.

When I need rejuvenation, I think of Tom. Three years after completing treatment with the first episode team, Tom came by to say hello and to ask how some of his old group members were doing. He had been a particularly difficult patient who was in restraints for seven days when I had originally joined the team. His denial had been rock hard, his compliance very poor, and his parents ready to send him packing with each relapse, of which there were three. It had been a long battle for him and he had attended many groups with me. When I told him how nice it was to see him, he said he thought it would be good for me to see how well he was doing. He said he knew that sometimes I worried about them (the group members). He could see it on my face. This day he wanted to cheer me up, he said, so I wouldn't give up on my clients. "I know sometimes we are very tough to work with." His timing was exquisite, better than mine ever could be. The latest recruits to the study were wearing me thin, at times making me feel hopeless. I needed the reminder that the hard work of group would eventually bear fruit. Six months later, Tom came by to say he was graduating from college and going to work as a counselor in a boy's school.

Tapping into the group's strength is a dynamic process, one that changes with the introduction of each new member. This means there is no clear set of rules for building a cohesive and therapeutic group. So what is it that I do in groups? I am still learning. I know I provide a feeling of safety. I provide structure and set limits. When necessary I help patients to connect with each other. I teach them about their illness. I facilitate the exploration of their ambivalence to treatment. I act as the group's organizing ego, but only as much as necessary. Then I step back and watch *the real healers* make magic.

REFERENCES

Freud, S. *On Beginning the Treatment. The Complete Psychological Works of Sigmund Freud.* London: Vol. 12, pp. 124-125, Hogarth Press, 1958.

Miller, R. and Mason, S. *So They Say I Have Schizophrenia.* New York: Columbia University Press (in press).

Miller, R. and Mason, S. (1998) Group Work with First Episode Schizophrenia Clients. *Social Work with Groups,* Vol 21 (1/2).

Yalom, I. (1995) *Theory and Practice of Group Psychotherapy.* 3rd ed. USA: Basic Books.